What If…

Everything you thought about stress is wrong?

Keep reading to learn why…

STRESS REIMAGINED

The Groundbreaking Way of Thinking and Dealing With Stress…

Carol L Rickard, LCSW

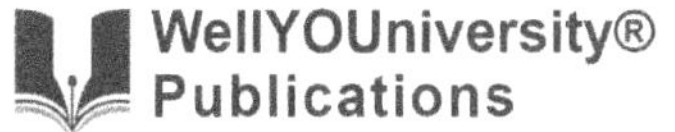

Stress REimagined

by Carol L Rickard, LCSW

ISBN: 978-1-947745-45-2 (paperback)
ISBN: 978-1-947745-46-9 (Ebook)

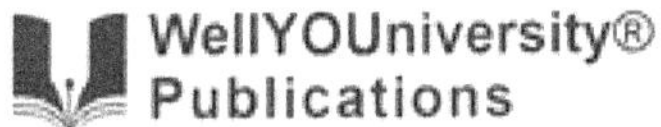

A Division of Well YOUniversity, LLC
5 Zion Rd.
Hopewell, NJ 08525
888 LIFE TOOLS (543-3866)
www.CarolRickard.com
Carol@CarolRickard.com

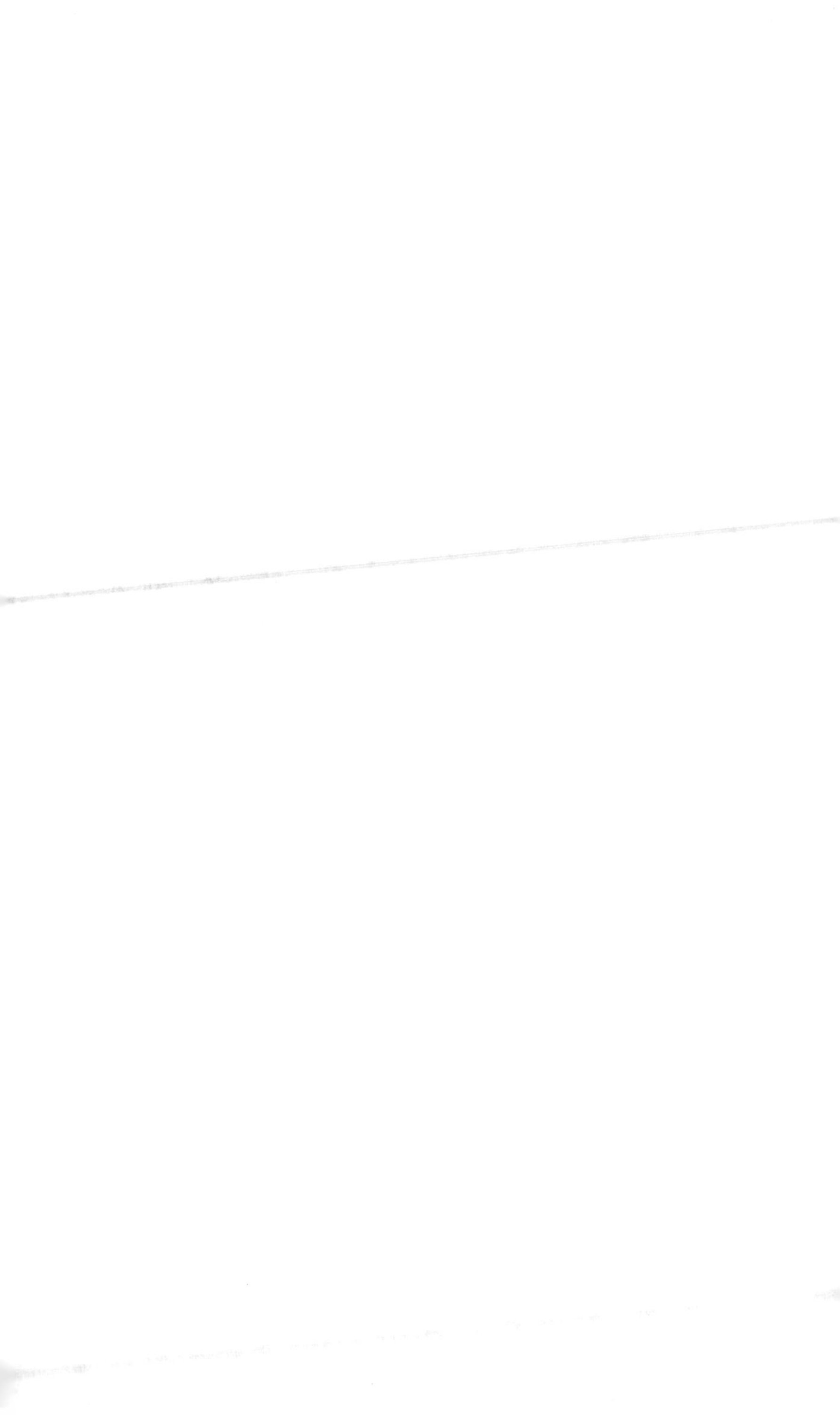

Could You

Be Living With

“Hidden Stress”?

Take the

“What’s Your Hidden Stress Risk?” Quiz

Tinyurl.com/HiddenQuiz

Contents

About This Book

I doubt you have read a  like this!

I like to use a lot of pictures, analogies, & word art which help information *stick* in the brain!

I call my approach:

***SMARTheory*™**

(It's what makes my books and trainings *different* from all others!)

KNOWLEDGE is the *left brain* at work.

This is where YOU ***know*** what to do!

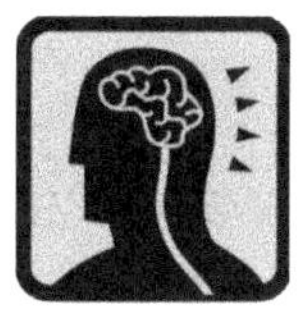

Since I use “pictures” & “images”, I end up

tapping into the other side of the brain –

the right side!

With both sides working

on the same page,

the result is getting people to

Move knowledge into ACTION!

This book is designed to be more like

“a workshop in a book”

So, you walk away with tools to use!

At What Cost?

***BEFORE* COVID** – stress could be found *all around the world* & already at **epidemic** levels -

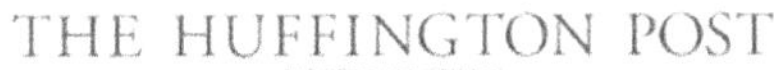

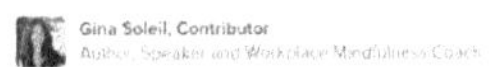

Workplace Stress: The Health Epidemic of the 21st Century

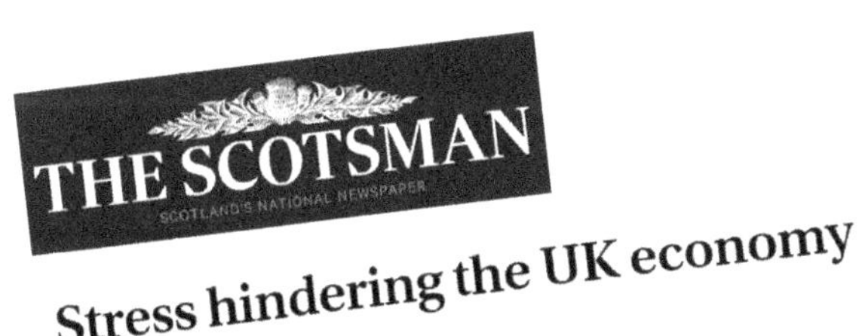
THE SCOTSMAN
SCOTLAND'S NATIONAL NEWSPAPER

Stress hindering the UK economy

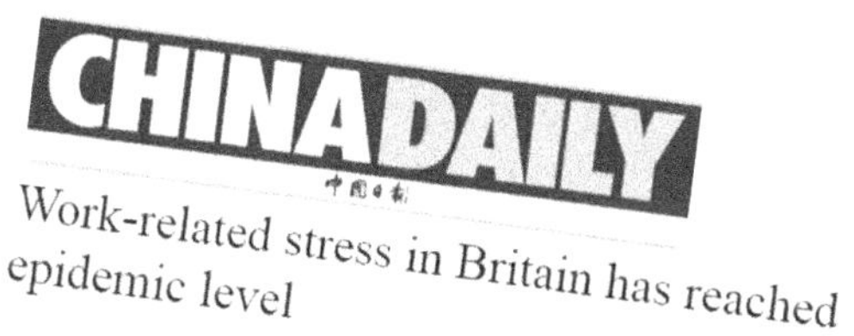
CHINA DAILY

Work-related stress in Britain has reached epidemic level

And **AFTER COVID…** (APA 2021-22 / *ALM 2021)

76%

Report stress has impacted their health.

48%

Say their behavior has been negatively affected by stress.

42%

Report gained more weight than they've intended.

23%

Say they are drinking more alcohol to cope with their stress.

$4.7 Billion a Week*

Estimated cost to US businesses / employers.

So, what does this mean?

Stress *is* even a **BIGGER** problem!

The  is:

What is stress **COSTING YOU?**

Are you so stressed out you can't sleep?

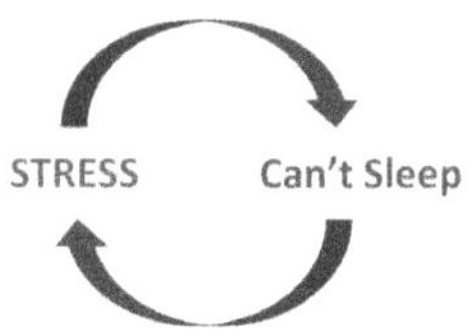

Is stress spilling out on the wrong people?

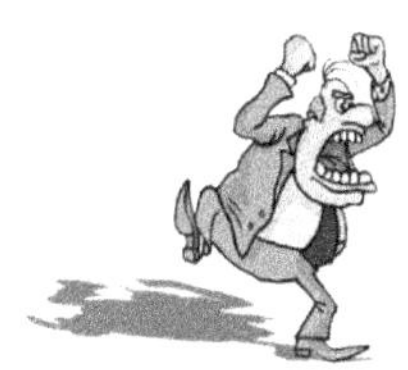
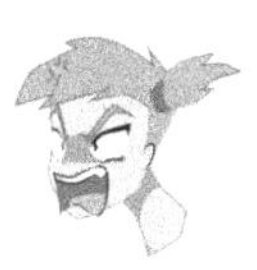
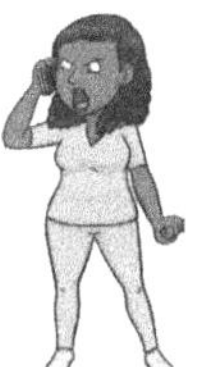

Are littlest things starting to get to you?

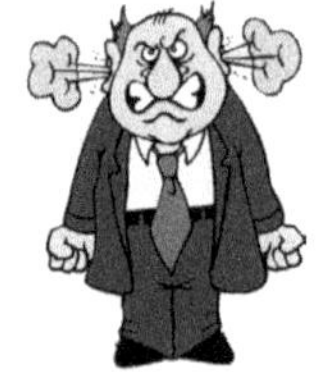

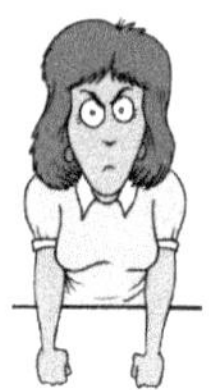

Do you get lost in overwhelm,
worry, or fear?

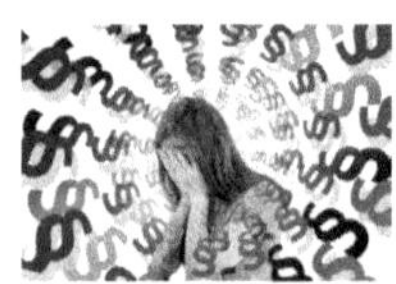
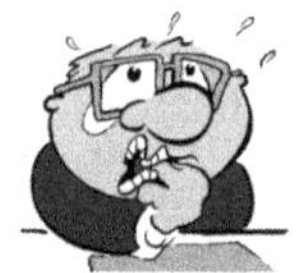

Are you experiencing anxiety,
depression, or sadness?

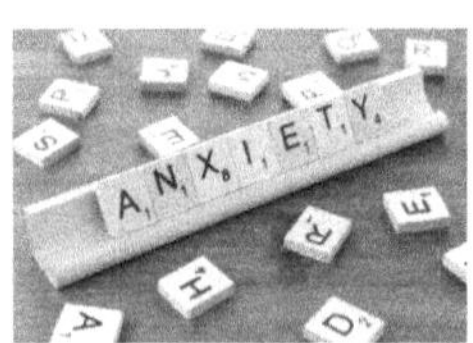

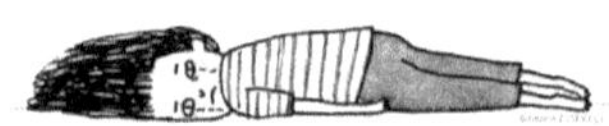
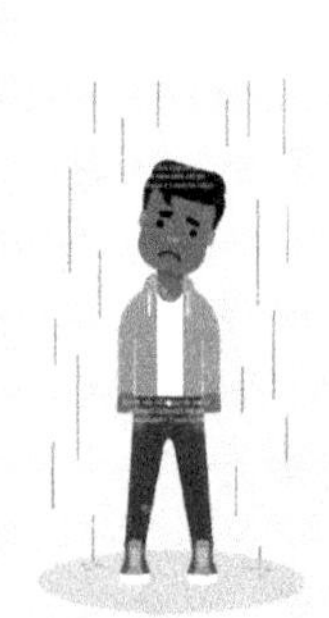

Are you having health issues?

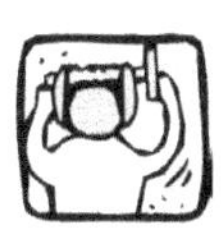

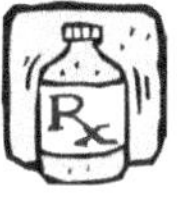

A "**yes**" to any of these is a sure sign

stress has *taken CONTROL* of your life.

Chances are...

no matter what you've tried it still

DOESN'T HELP.

And it's *not your fault*. Here's why.....

What *we've been taught*

Isn't Working!

(Keep reading & find out why 😊 !)

The problem…

when **Stress** is not controlled,

it has the *power to ruin* a lot of things…

sleep

health

relationships

families

&… careers.

It is my sincere hope you will take

what you learn in this book &

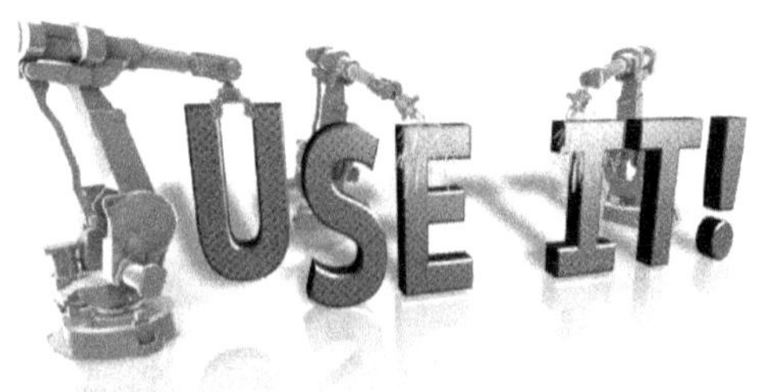

The best way to get a sense of

how things ***are for you*** is

to track your **Stress Quotient**

Using the scale below,

what is your average daily stress level?

10 - 100

Low High

Write it in here:

My guarantee to you:

If you will use what is in this

you will *at least* **cut that level in 1/2.**

Don't Miss This SPECIAL Offer!

Join Carol for the

Stress Smarter Masterclass

This 45-minute video training with Carol is a quick way to reinforce what you're learning!

ONLY $7

For A Limited Time…

SAVE $140

Tinyurl.com/bycarol

A New Way

Making Stress Visible

Imagine –

I'm standing in front of you,

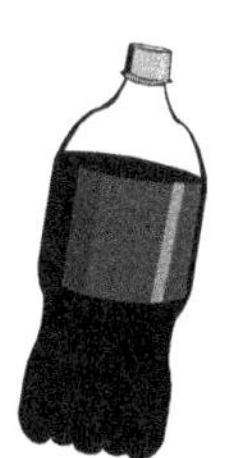

holding a big bottle of root beer.

*I SHAKE it up… **a lot,***

then I drop it on the floor twice!

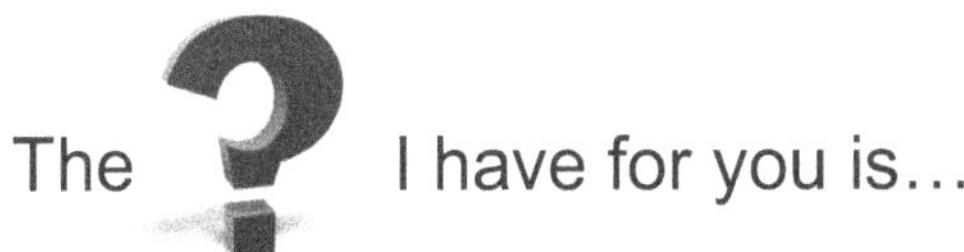

The ? I have for you is…

Do you **want** to open it?

If you're like *99%* of my clients,

You'll say:

" **NO –** It's going to **Explode!** "

RIGHT! The pressure built up inside.

People are just like bottles of root beer…

Life happens every day that

shakes us up!

…from the moment we wake up the

PRESSURE

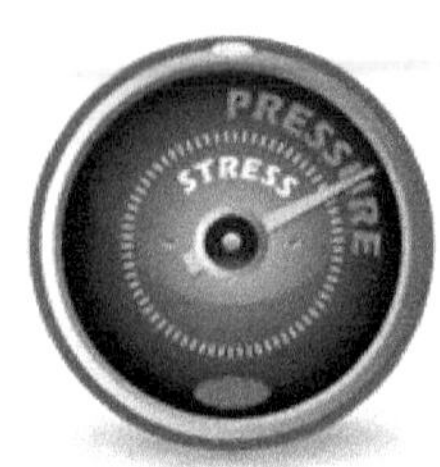

builds up *inside us!*

For some: it starts the night before!

However, unlike the bottle…

People can **ONLY**

hold so much…

before they do one of 3 things:

#1 – EXPLODE

It comes ***spilling out***

on the wrong person or

at the wrong time.

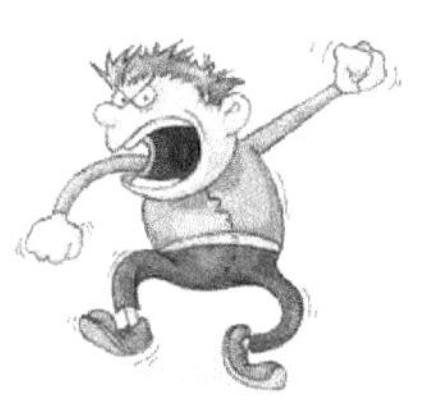

#2 – IMPLODE

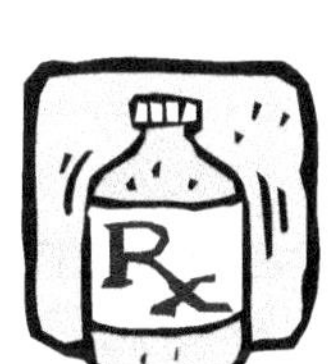

It ***stays inside***,

& makes ***them*** sick.

#3 – COMBO

Hold in 95% time, but

it then **spills out** usually

on 1 person or 1 situation.

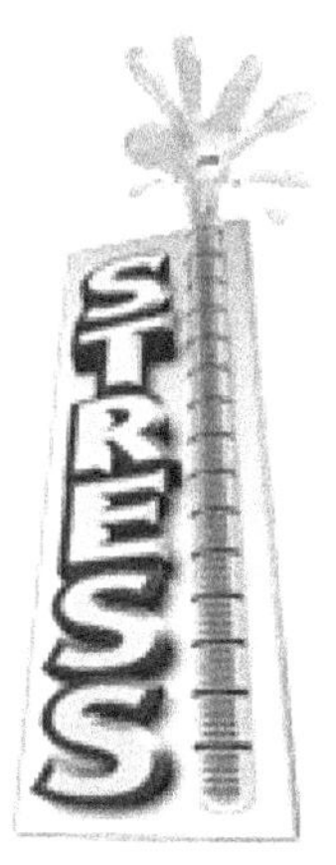

Which of those ***best*** describes you?

Circle your answer below:

#1
Explode

#2
Implode

#3
Combo

IMPORTANT:

It's **NOT** *your fault* this is happening.

This all happens at an *unconscious level*

& will continue until we **change it.**

There's…

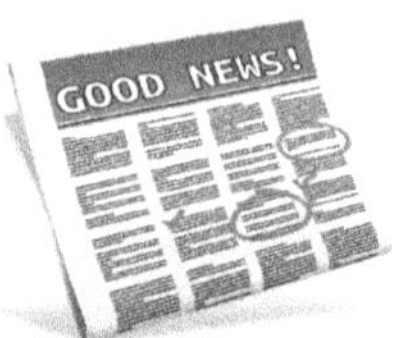

You
CAN
change
this!

A Critical Point

Once that pressure gets

BUILT UP in the bottle…

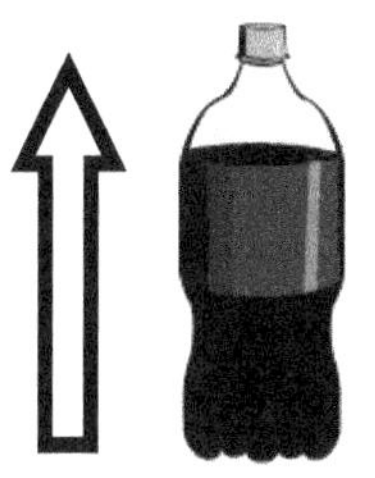

IT STAYS THERE

until it is released!

Same thing happens to people!

Our **STRESS**

doesn't go anywhere

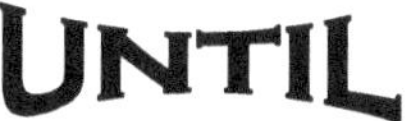

we *let it out!*

MOST people hold it in for years

leading to… **Burnout**

Seeing It Another Way

Imagine…

Turning on the water in your tub at 9:00am

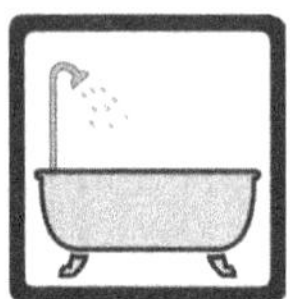

And then not going back to shut it off

UNTIL 6:00 pm that night….

What do you think you'd come back to?

A MESS!

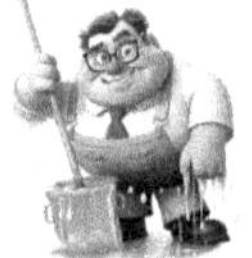

Unfortunately,

this happens to *millions of people…*

At the end of their days

They end up **A STRESS MESS!**

22 years ago, *I was that mess!*

When I started my dream job at the

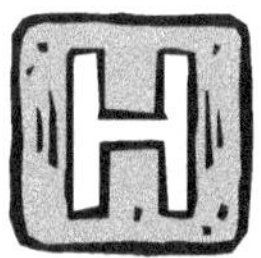

STRESS took ***control*** of me!

Only…

I didn't *realize* it at the time…

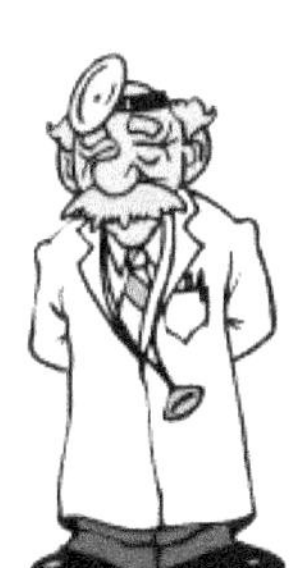

It wasn't until I landed

in my doctor's office

3 weeks in a row

with a ***horrible migraine*** & he asked

(MY IMPLOSION)

"Carol, what's got you so stressed?"

The **embarrassing** part -

I worked in a hospital *teaching*

stress management

& here's my doctor's telling me

I'm not doing a very good job myself.

But ***I was*** doing EVERYTHING I taught:

- I was exercising. 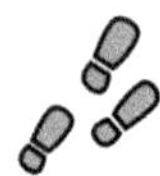
- Trying to eat healthy. 
- Spending time with family & friends.
- And even volunteering. 

The Problem...

My work was ***so stressful…***

my stress would build up

& by 2:00 o'clock in the day

I'd end up with another

horrible migraine.

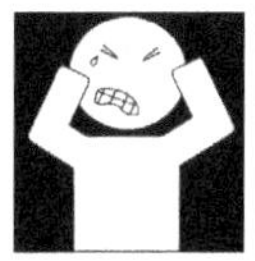

Desperate To Not Get Fired And End the Migraines...

I decided to start using some of

the ***"tools"*** I was teaching for

just 60 *seconds*

throughout my day.

Most times,

it was ***only 10 or 15 seconds*** because

I was super busy with patients.

My hope was if I could keep my stress

level from getting so ***HIGH*** at work,

it would make a difference.

And it did…

That following week was the 1st time

in a month I didn't get a migraine

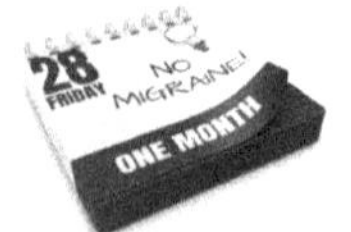

and leave work early.

I kept using my system

over the next few months

with the same **amazing result:**

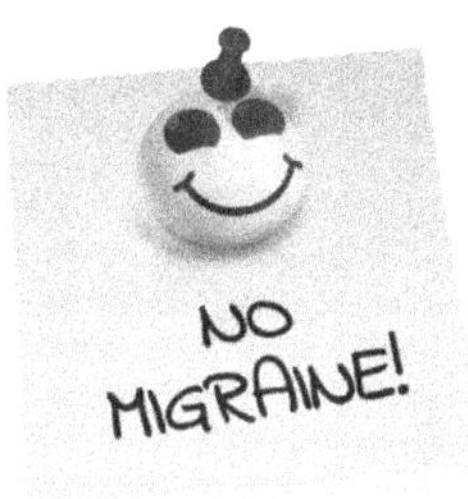

Curious to find out if it was just a fluke,

I ***began teaching this*** to the

patients and staff at the hospital.

And to my surprise,

They too started having great success!

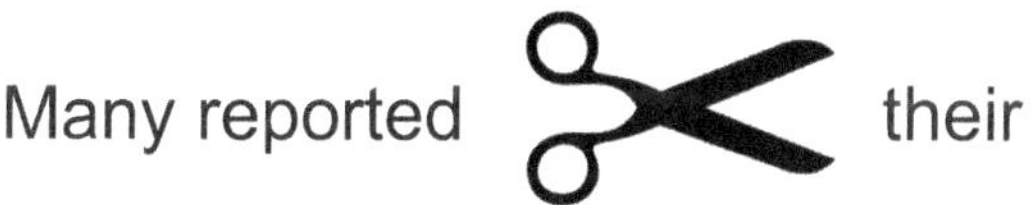
Many reported ✂ their

stress & anxiety levels in ½!

That's when I realized I'd discovered

A 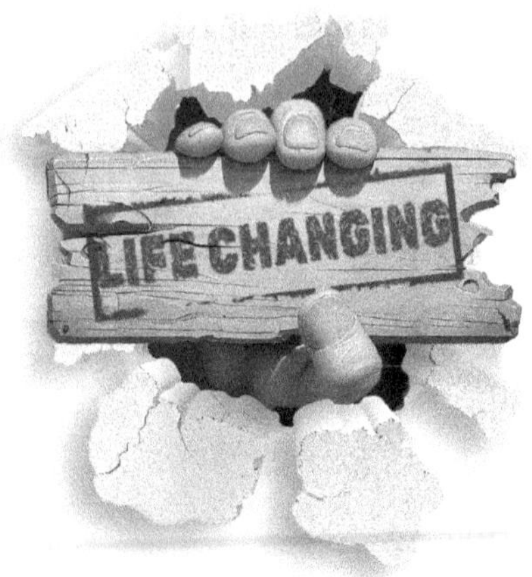

Method!

That when we use…

*the **right tools** in the **right order**,*

we can take control of stress & anxiety

anytime, anywhere in just seconds!

I call this life-changing discovery:

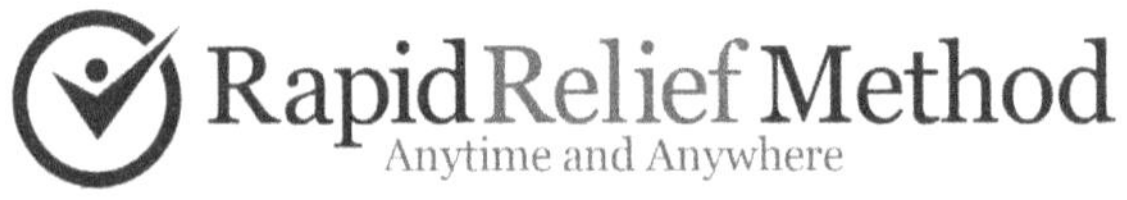

Since then…

I've gone on to teach

this method & the tools to

1,000's across the world

&

many top organizations including:

STATE
POLICE
NJ

PRINCETON
UNIVERSITY

PHL
PHILADELPHIA
INTERNATIONAL AIRPORT

SEPTA

U.S. DEPARTMENT OF
ENERGY

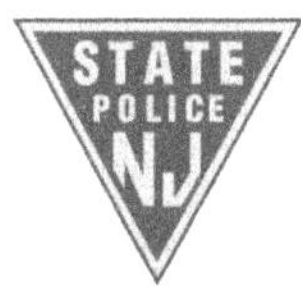

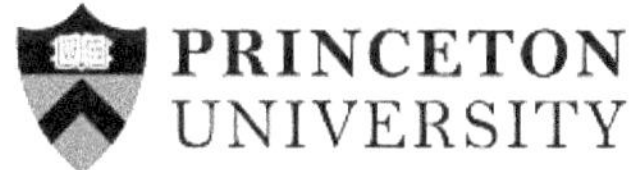

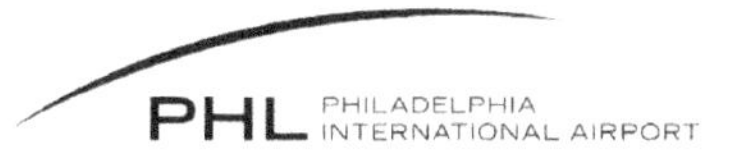

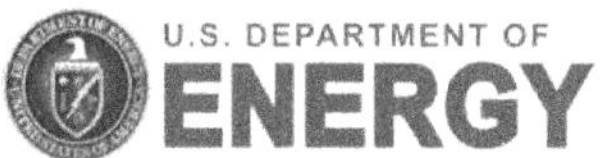

I've also been a featured in various media:

Reader's
digest

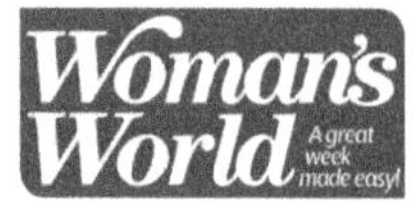

DR.OZ
THE GOOD LIFE

Today…

I am so grateful for the chance

to teach it to you!

How It Works!

Could You

Be Living With

"Hidden Stress"?

Take the

"What's Your Hidden Stress Risk?" Quiz

Tinyurl.com/HiddenQuiz

What Is Stress?

STRESS is…

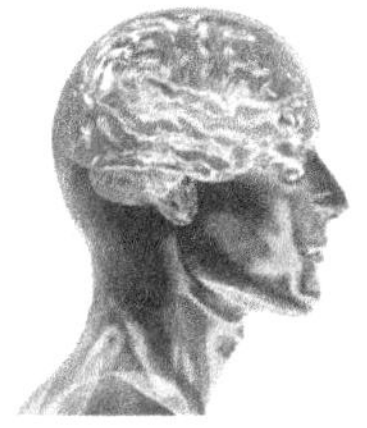

Our
Brain's
Survival
Mechanism

It is going **24** *hours a day*

& you CAN'T STOP THE PROCESS!

It's hardwired to respond to

changes or situations

to keep us alive!

It's kind of like your car alarm…

It's ALWAYS running!

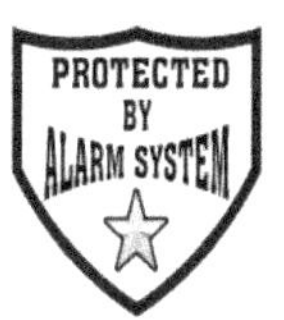

However, recent research has proven we

CAN *TAKE CONTROL* of this process.

It all starts with…

using the RIGHT

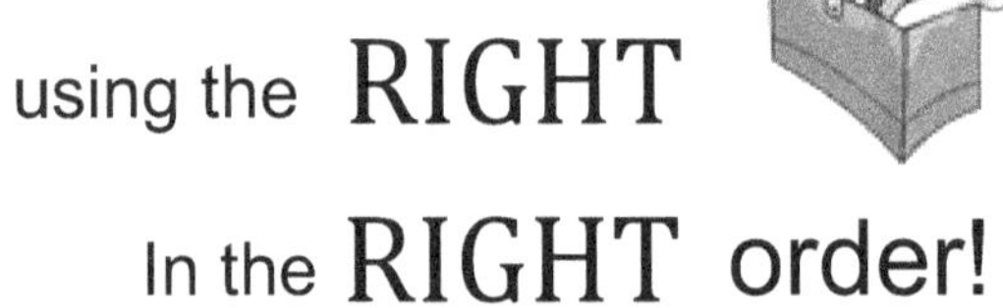

In the RIGHT order!

Now…

Think about how many

changes or situations

you face in just one day?

A LOT!

FYI! *STRESS* comes wrapped

in ***a lot of different packages…***

Stress can be…

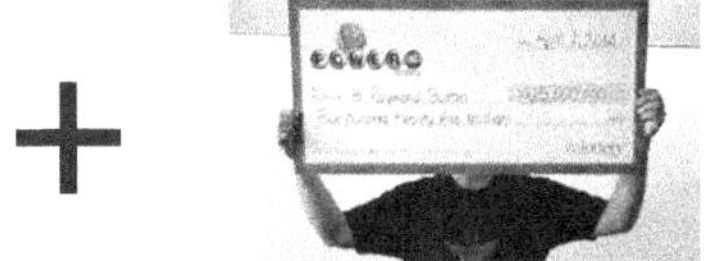

Winning $400 million Powerball! *(I wish!)*

or

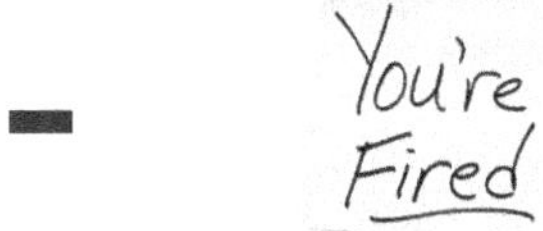

Getting terminated from my job.

It can also be a…

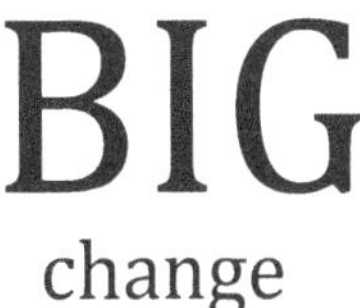

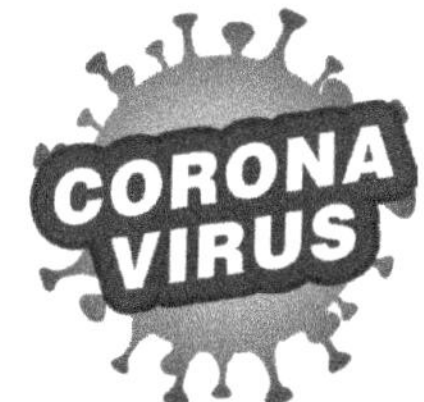

or

SMALL
change

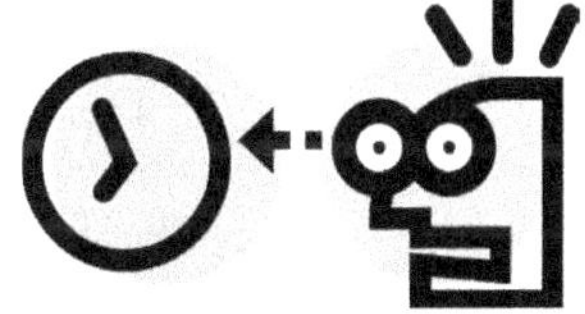

Leaving 2 minutes late!

Lastly,

Changes & situations can be either…

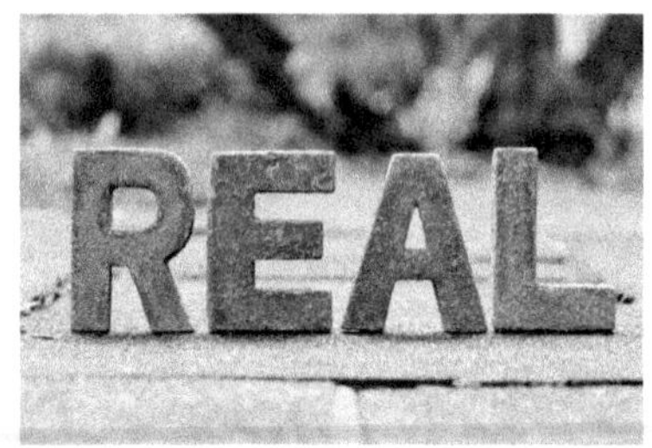

They exist!

or

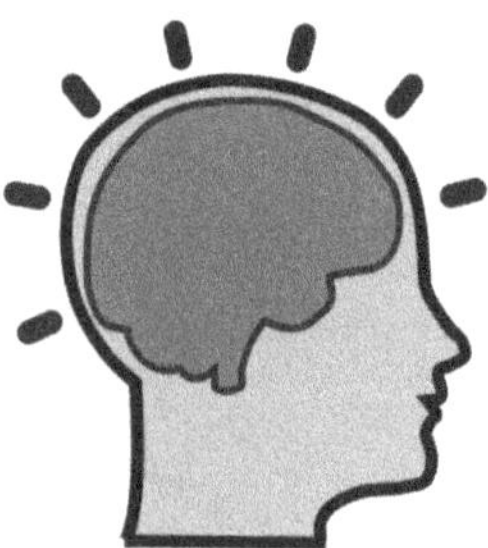

Just a thought in our mind!

When it comes to stress - our brain has

3 basic responses…

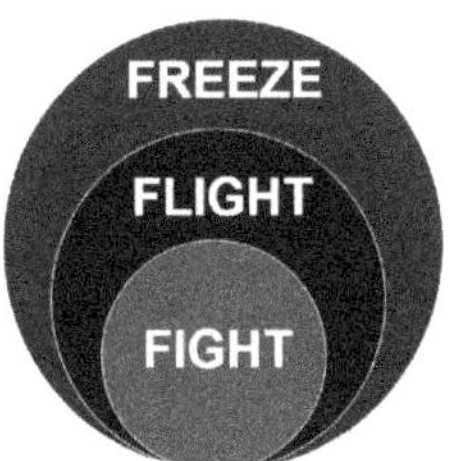

But there's one more I've uncovered

during my **30+** year career...

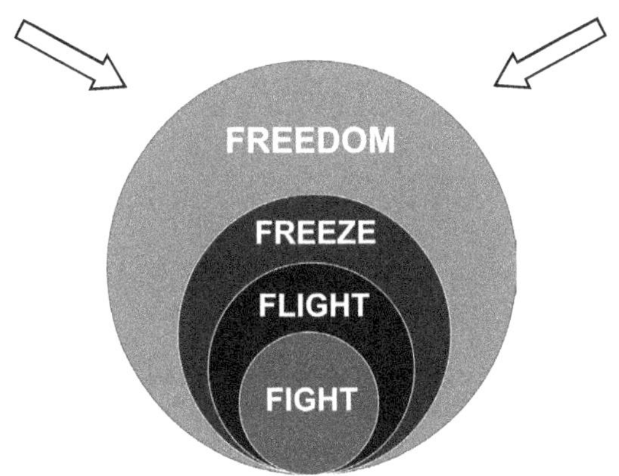

Taking action

stress no longer <u>negatively</u> <u>impacts</u> us!

Brainology 101!

Our brain has a built in "*alarm system*",

I call it: **The Defense Center.**

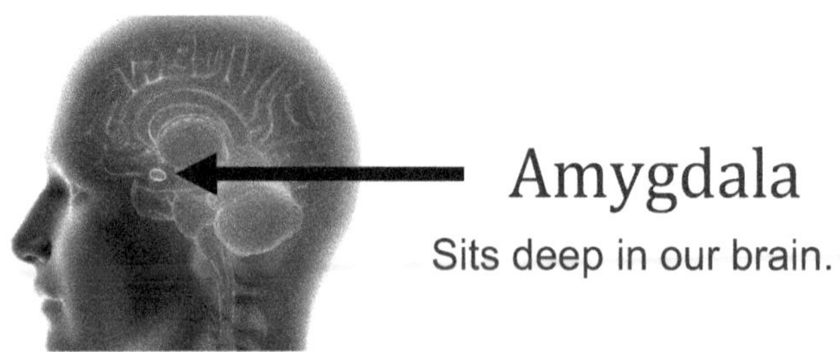

It's *constantly* operating &

scanning our **environment**

for what it perceives as potential threats:

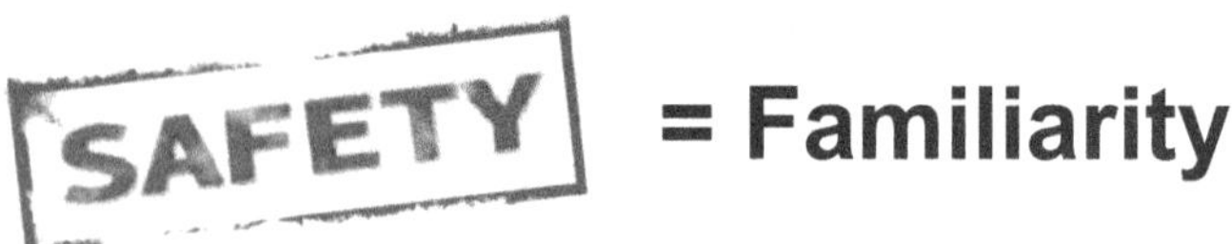

Our brains…

like things to stay the same!

When it detects a change or a

situation it's not familiar with…

It sounds the alarm!

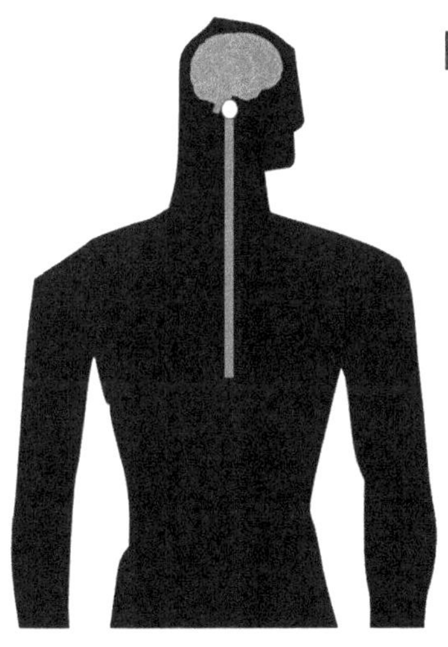

Defense Center

sends signals

& *energy to*

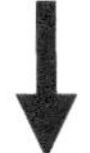

Our Body

We can't stop this –

Only MANAGE IT!

And our "stress response" is turned on to:

Fight

Flight

Freeze

Here's an example…

Has this ever **happened** to you?

It's the night before

you leave for…

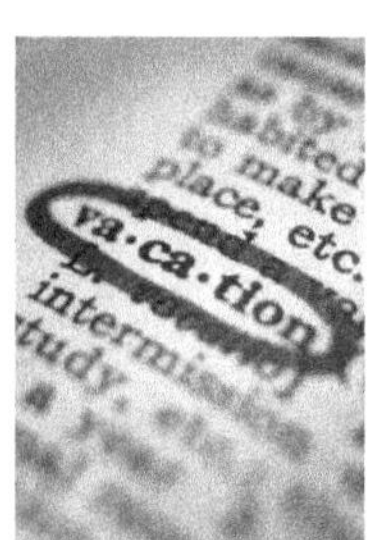

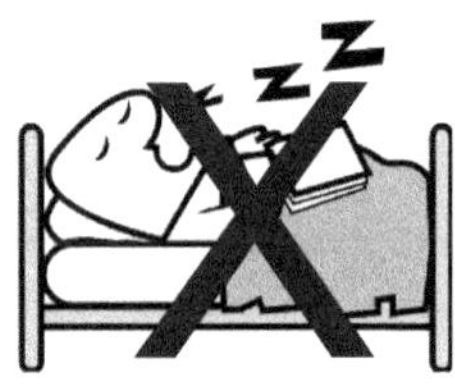

And You

CAN'T sleep!

That's because your brain

is ***responding to the*** **CHANGE**

happening the next morning!

Using the

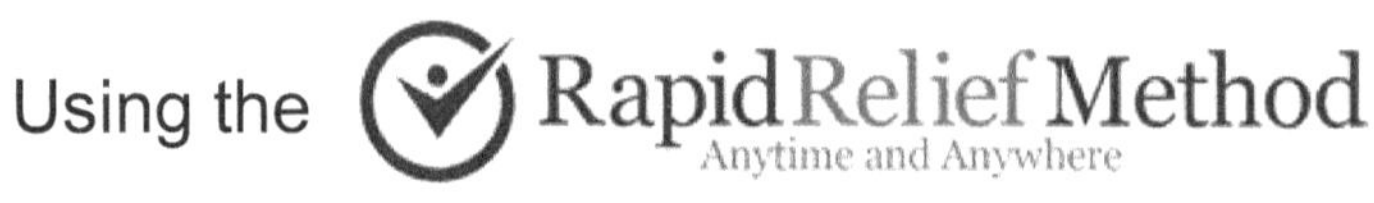

You'll be able to get some sleep!

A better way to think of
this process is to
come back to our tub!

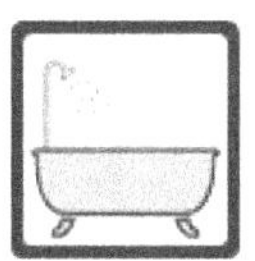

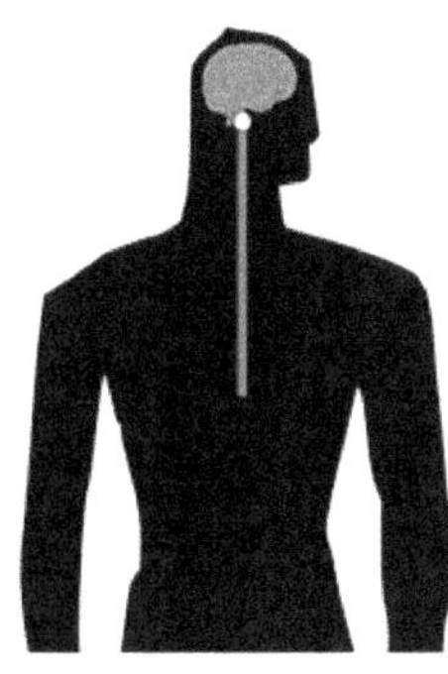

The Brain = Faucet

The Body = Tub

And a tub can only hold so much before it:

OVERFLOWS!

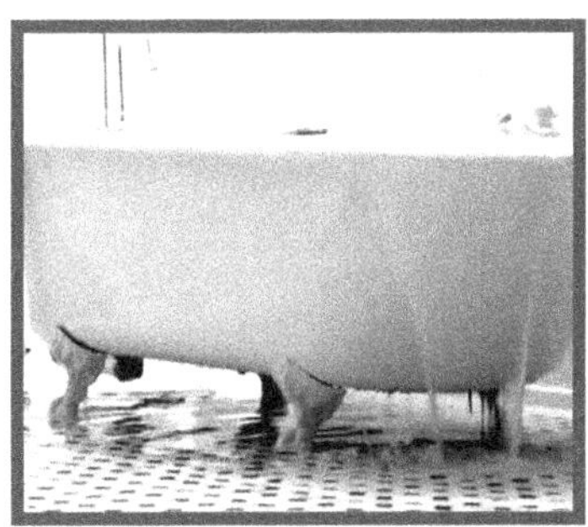

Why Is Stress Good?

Has this ever ***happened*** to you?

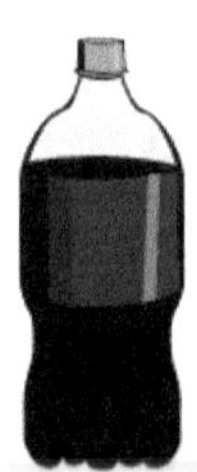

You're looking forward to a nice

cold root beer (or seltzer)…

You go to take a sip and

UGHHHHHH – it's *completely* **FLAT!**

Would you agree…

A little bit of PRESSURE is actually

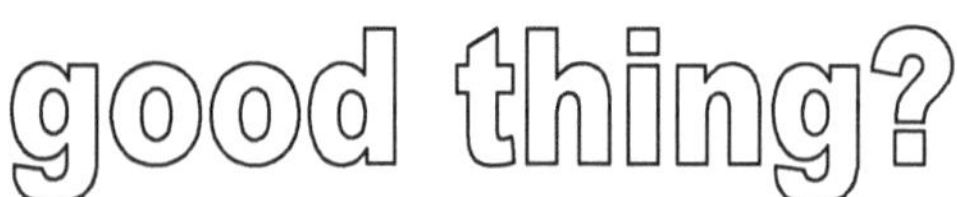

The same holds true about stress.

A little bit is a GOOD THING…

The key with both:

Having the **RIGHT** AMOUNT!

In fact,

Research shows how moderate ***short term* stress** has very positive benefits:

✓ ⇧ Performance 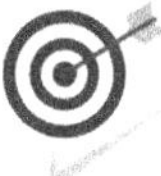

✓ ⇧ Immunity 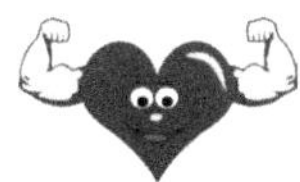

✓ ⇧ Brain Power 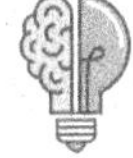

✓ ⇧ Motivation 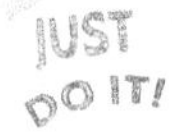

KEY: It all comes down to having an

OPTIMAL *level…*

An "Optimal Level" looks like this:

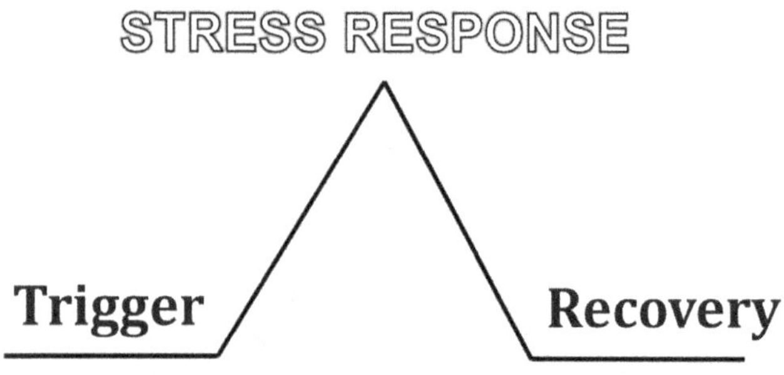

The **"stress response"** gets triggered

& then can ***recover.***

In other words…

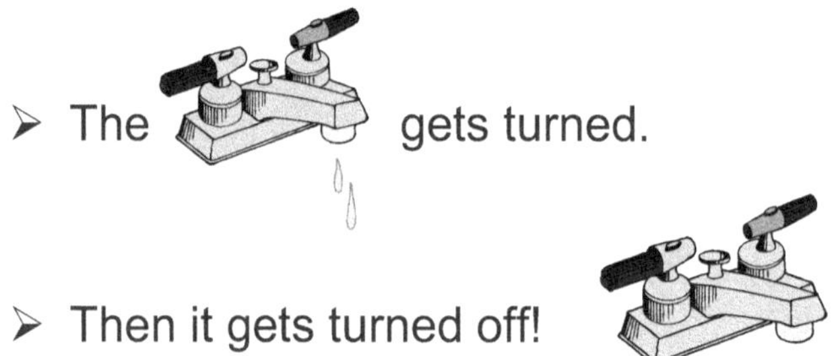

- The [faucet] gets turned.
- Then it gets turned off!
- And the level in the tub subsides.

But in today's world…

most people are like this:

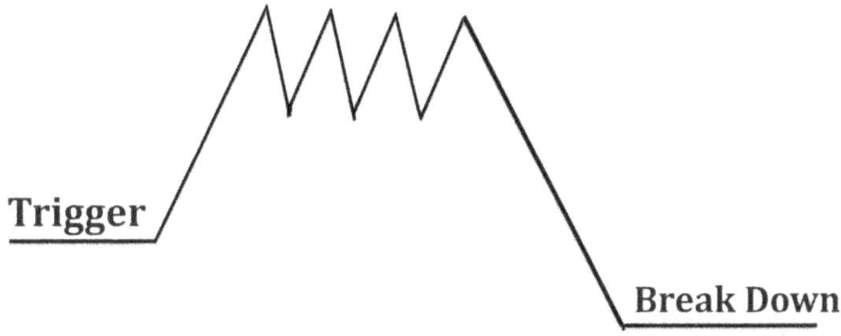

In other words…

- The 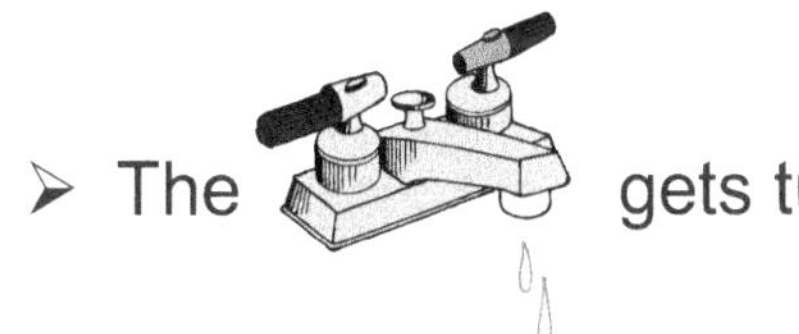 gets turned on.
- It **NEVER** gets turned off. 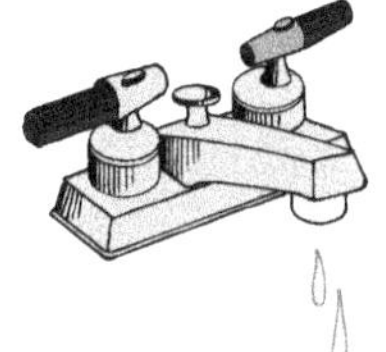
- The tub **OVERFLOWS!** 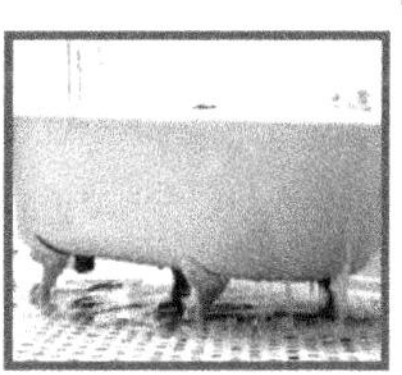

The KEY to success is to

recognize your stress level's

***BUILDING* too high** 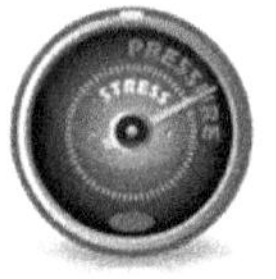

& do something

to RELEASE IT…

BEFORE you

Explode

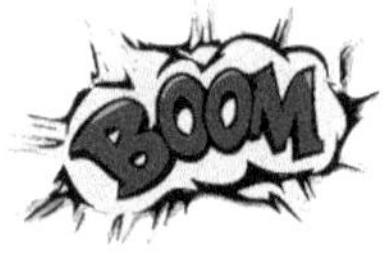

Implode

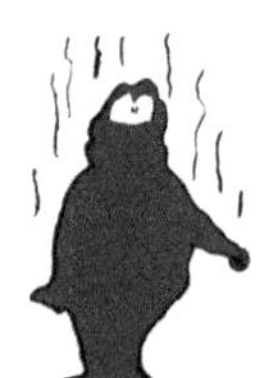

Combo

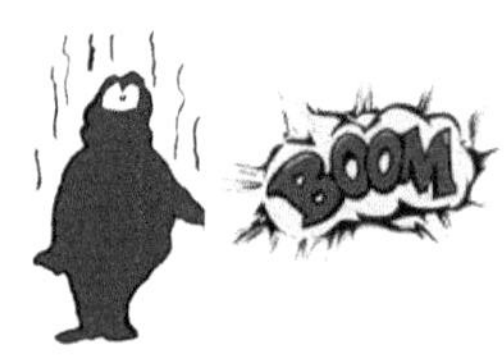

Let's look at what you can do to change things!

Take Control!

Could You

Be Living With

"Hidden Stress"?

Take the

"What's Your Hidden Stress Risk?" Quiz

Tinyurl.com/HiddenQuiz

The Right Tools

What is the **only** thing that will

take out Superman?

KRYPTONITE!

When it comes to stress, we all have…

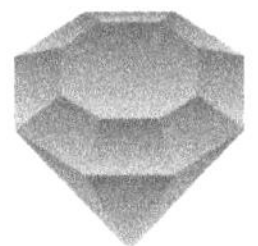

Stress Kryptonite!

Science is very clear…

the fastest way to STOP our

stress response is *breathe…*

HOW ***you do it*** MATTERS.

There are a few ways

I want you to practice with me.

Do this test with me…

Put **1** hand on your chest &

one hand on your belly like this:

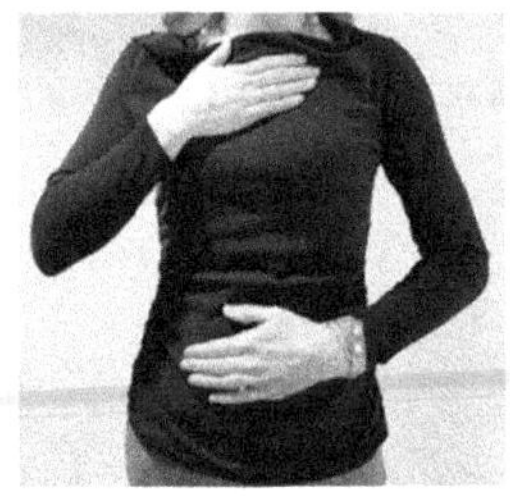

Take a breath & **NOTICE**
which hands moves.

(You might need to repeat this a couple times to be sure!)

I'm afraid I have some bad news if…

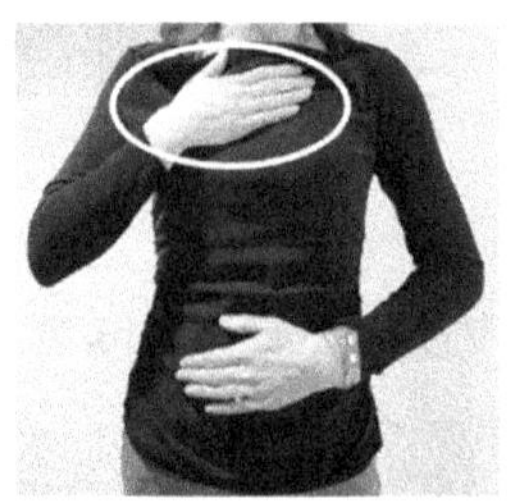

this hand *MOVED.*

This *won't work!*

We ***need*** to get air into

the <u>bottom part</u> of our lungs…

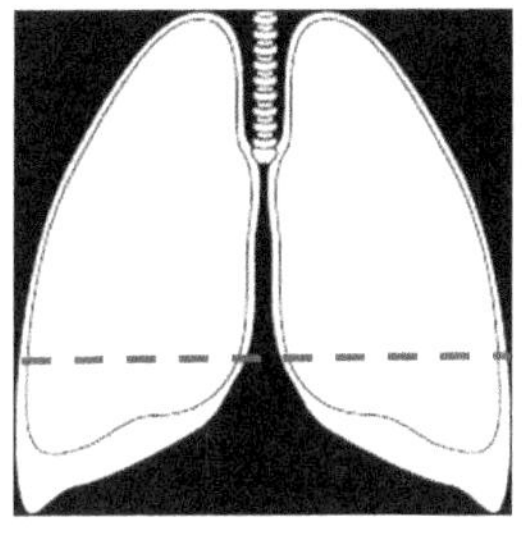

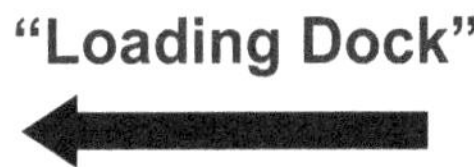

This is where oxygen gets

"loaded" into our bloodstream!

It's like this…..

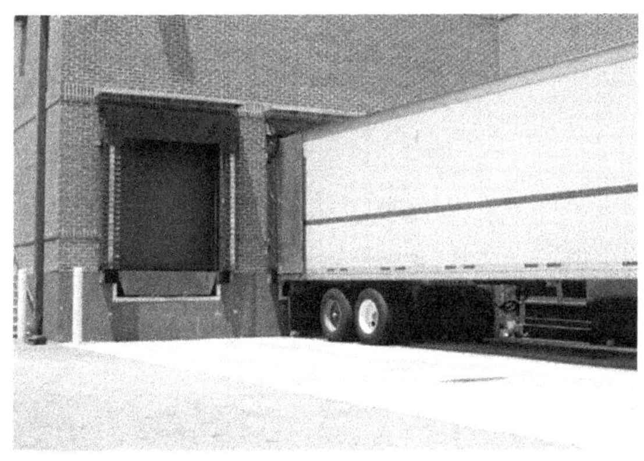

Versus…

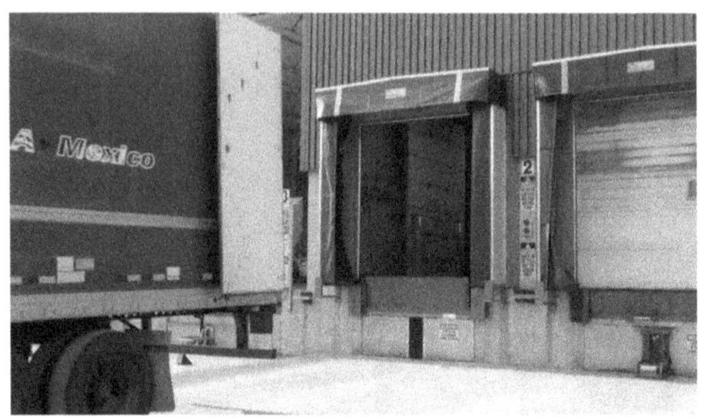

So,

Let's try this again BUT this time,

concentrate on making

the hand on your belly move!

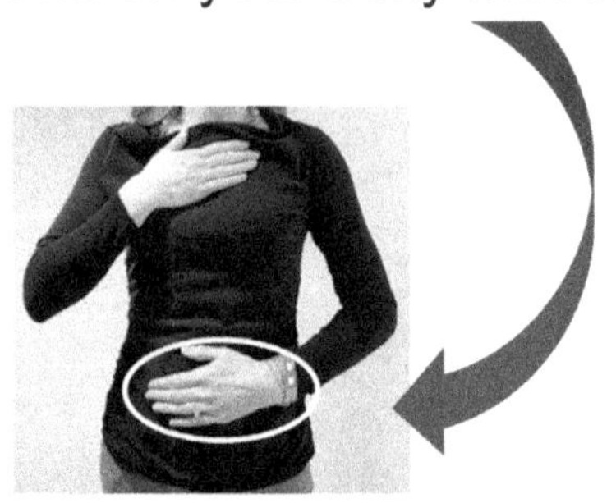

Ready? 1,2,3…*BREATHE*

Don’t worry

If you don’t get it *right away,*

it’s something that needs **PRACTICE!**

A good way to do this:

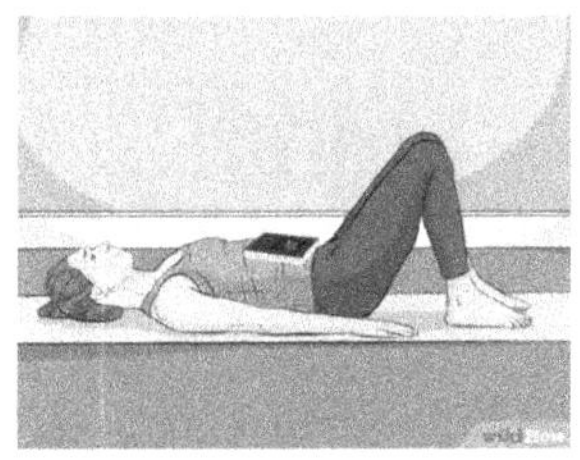

As you breathe in,
try to *raise the book!*

Have you ever watched a 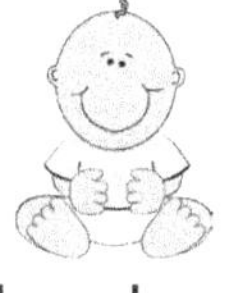 sleep?

What ***MOVES*** when they breathe?

Right!!!! Their belly!

Here’s the thing…

We’re all born **“belly breathers”** –

Somewhere along the way *we* ***changed.***

I have a theory...

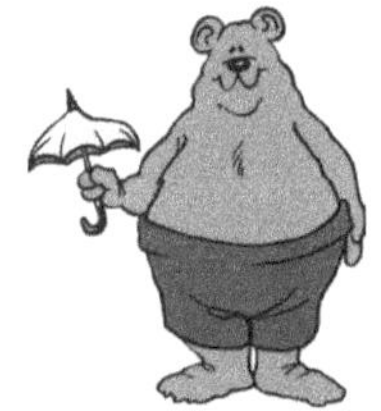

When our clothes started

to fit a ***little tighter*****.....**

we started *sucking the air* up **higher!**

Have you ever heard that

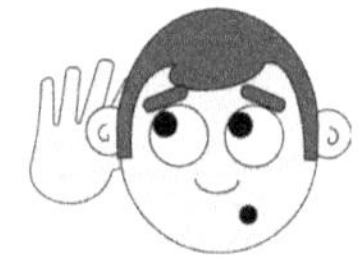

Belly Breathing

&

Yoga Breathing

are ***good for our health***?

This is WHY!

S l o w i n g our *breathing*

will also 

our stress response!

When **stress pressure** starts building up -

our **breathing** *starts*

SPEEDING UP!

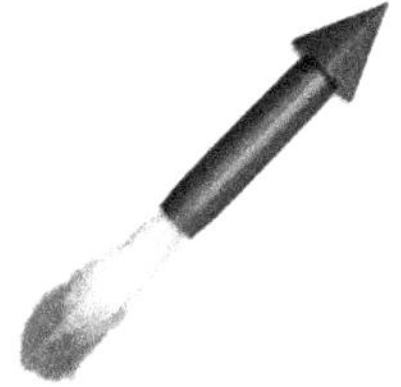

It's part of the brain's **"HARD WIRING"**

designed to keep us alive!

Taking control of our breath

as you inhale & exhale

helps **OVERRIDE**

the stress response.

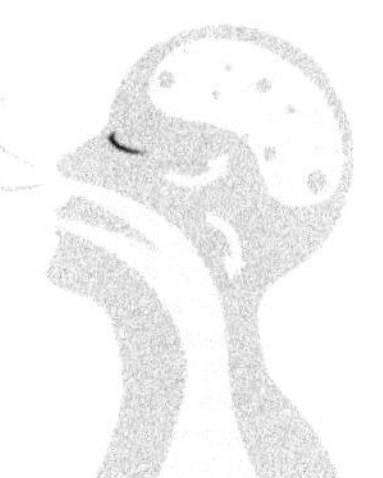

The RESET Breath

This is another breathing tool

backed by scientific research. 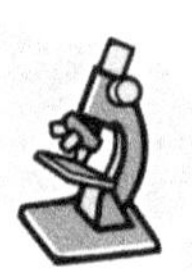

Do this with me **right now** –

Breathe IN:

(thru the nose) S L O W

count of 5

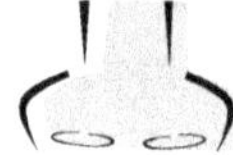

Breathe OUT:

(thru the mouth) ***S L O W E R***

count of 7

Do 3 Breaths!

Here's how it works…

When we SLOW DOWN our breathing,

Our 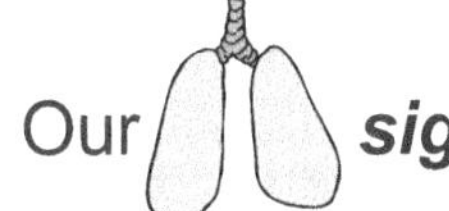 ***signal our heart*** to slow down.

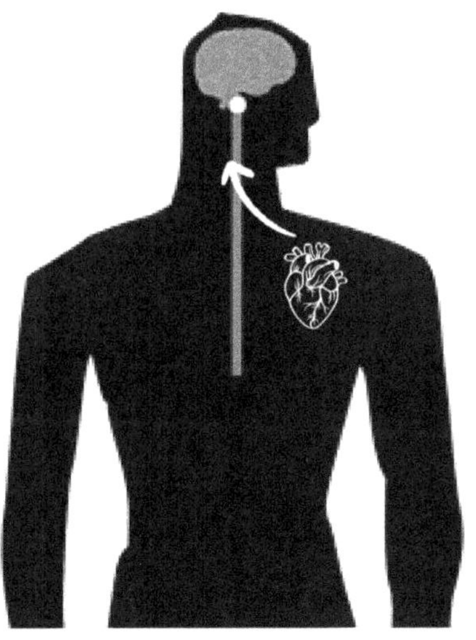

Our heart then ***signals our brain*** to

turn off the stress faucet!

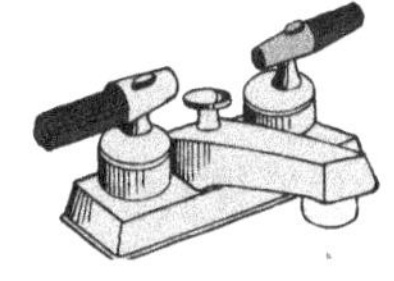

The CALM Switch

1 more breathing tool I want

to share is what's known as

the ***"physiological sigh"***.

Science has proven this is the

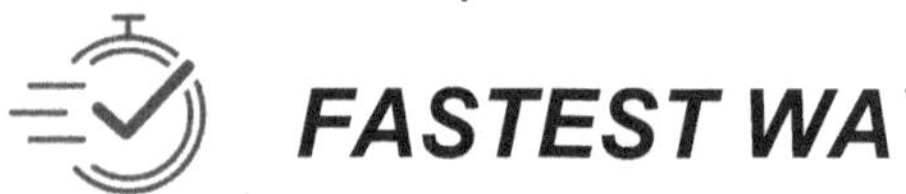

to "turn off our stress faucet"!

P.S. We all do this

when we're sleeping.

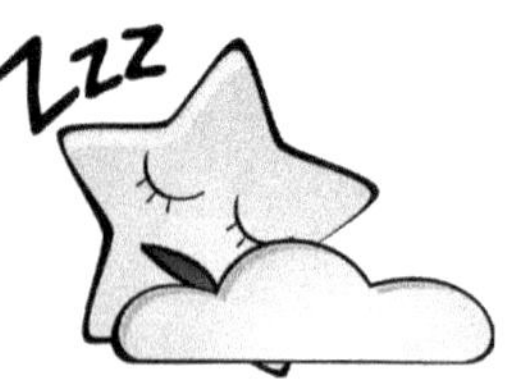

Even just 1 breath works!

Go to: **Tinyurl.com/TheCalmSwitch**

Here's how to do it –

Breathe IN:

(thru the nose)

For a count of 3

½ Way Thru:

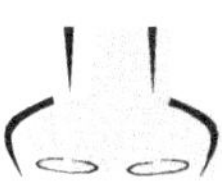

Take another ***QUICK*** breath in - (like a snort!)

Breathe OUT:

(thru the mouth)

S L O W

count of 6

Use the video to help you practice…

Tinyurl.com/TheCalmSwitch

Dump n Destroy

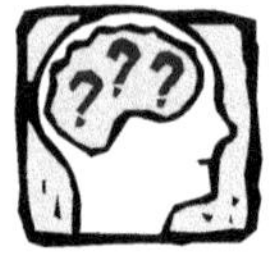

This is one of my ***secret weapons***!

Here's what you need:

- ✓ A piece of paper
- ✓ Something to write with

1) Simply **Start** *writing*

2) ***DO NOT*** READ IT

3) ***Destroy*** *IT!*

It's **very** different from "Journaling"

which can be another great tool!

PS. *You* ***CANNOT*** *use a computer or phone!*

The goal is to just *get it out…*

When you **read it**, you **RELOAD** it!

It *doesn't* make problems go away.

It DOES give

moments **of relief.**

If ***you're afraid*** someone will *read it* -

Try this…

The Disappearing Dump!

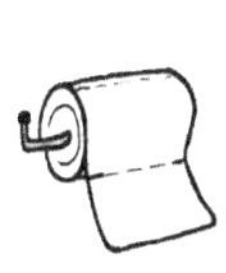

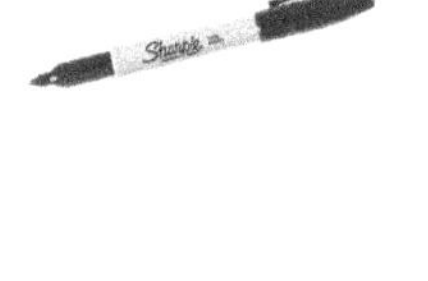

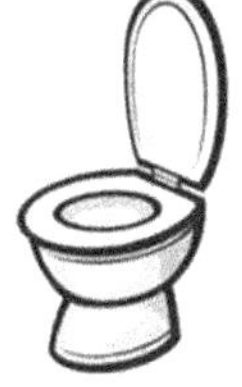

- **Go in the bathroom**
- **"Dump" on toilet paper**
- **Flush it when done!**

Variations:

#1 - Dealing with Loss

This is my ***dearest*** friend who passed…

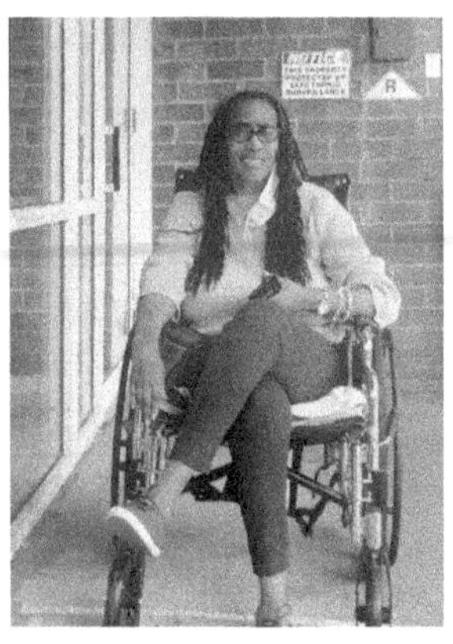

Hope Taylor

Nov. 2020

Honor Book

- Get a journal
- Put a loved one's photo on the front
- Write a letter to them as often as you like as if you were talking with them.

It's an *IMPORTANT* way

to **honor & release** the feelings.

#2 - Not Sure What You're Feeling

This is a great way to *Dump N Destroy*

when you're just **not sure**

WHAT you're feeling or thinking

(or you'll try to ***read*** what you write!)

Here's what to do:

- ✓ Get a piece of paper
- ✓ Grab markers, crayons, pastels
- ✓ Pick colors that match your feeling

Here's a few examples of one of my clients:

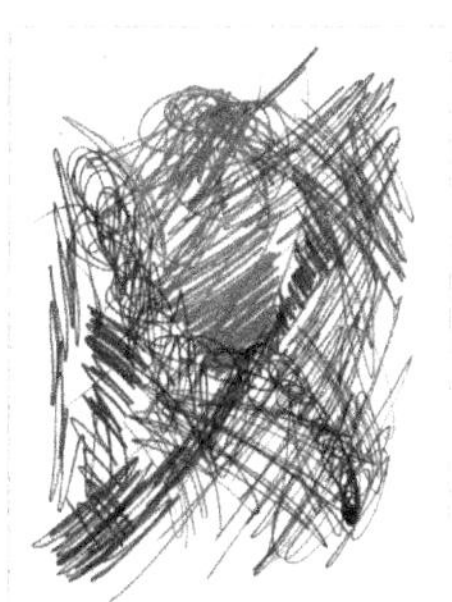

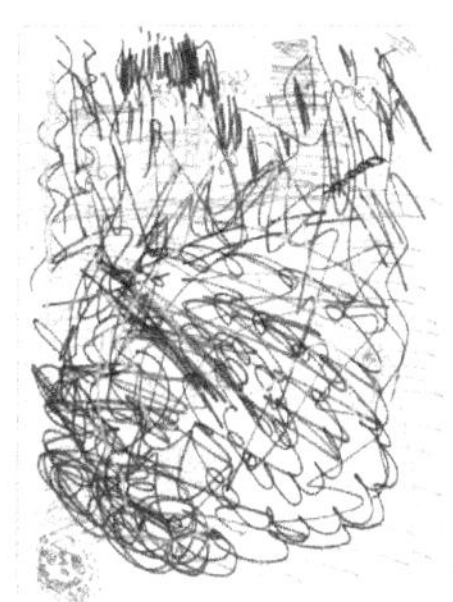

#3 - Can't Shut Off The Mind

It also works *really well* when…

1) You can't **fall asleep** because your *mind racing*

2) You **wake up** at night & your mind is racing!

**IMPORTANT:

You must go write in ***another*** room for it to work.

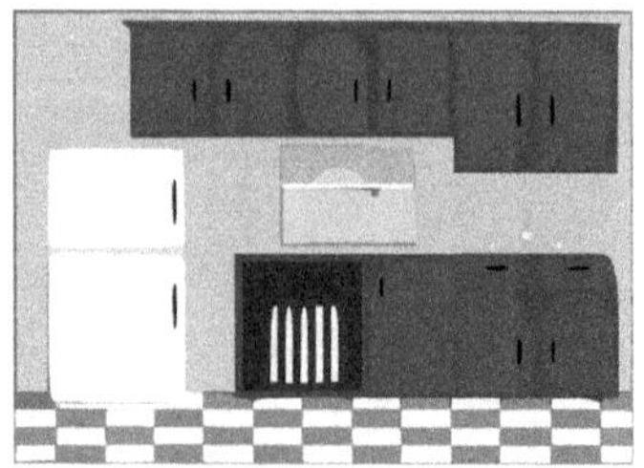

The kitchen is a good place to do this!

Don't turn on any overhead lights.

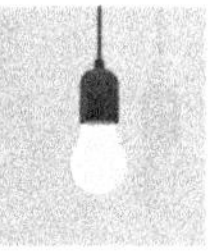

(You don't want to wake your brain up!)

Instead,

Use the **stove** light or a **night** light.

Here's what to do:

- ✓ Go to kitchen
- ✓ ***Dump*** on notepad
- ✓ DO NOT READ it
- ✓ Go back & lay down

Don't be surprised if you *must repeat!*

(You may have ***A LOT to dump!***)

When you wake up –

If it's "crap" from the day before – ***destroy***

If it's stuff for the day to come – *USE IT!*

#4 - Anytime, Anywhere!

There's 1 more variation!

NO PAPER NEEDED...

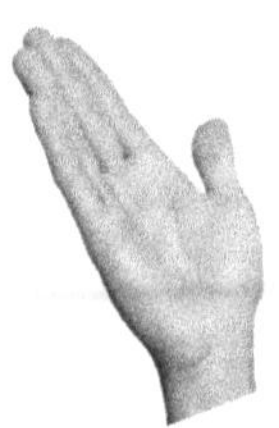

Your hand = **PAPER**

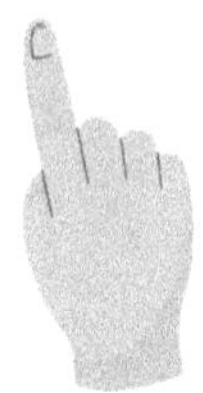

Your finger = **PEN**

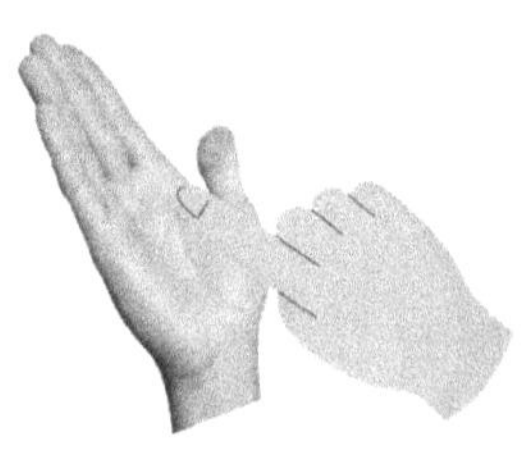

DUMP!

When done – blow it away!

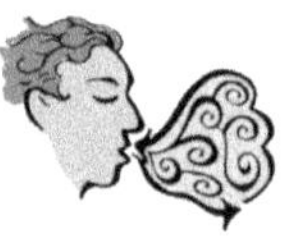

Mind Push-Ups

One last **RIGHT TOOL:**

"Mind Pushup's"!

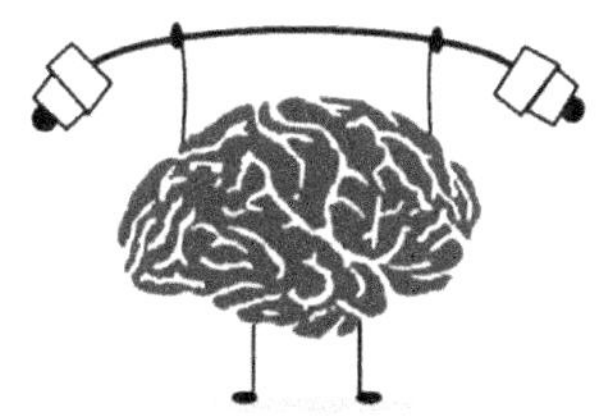

I used to think I ***couldn't meditate***

because my mind wouldn't be **QUIET!**

That was until...

I met a Buddhist Tibetan Nun who taught

me what I'm about to teach you!

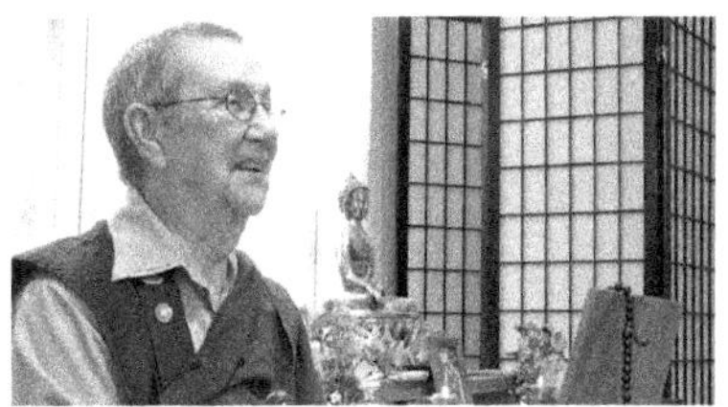

My teacher:

Ani Trime

She explained there are

4,000 types of meditation!

“I’m going to teach you the simplest one:”

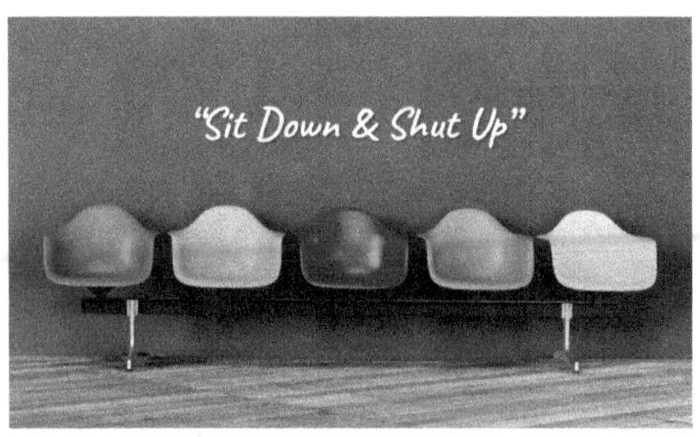

I remember thinking to myself -

‘I can do that!’

The goal of **Mind Push-Up’s** is to:

STRENGTHEN OUR

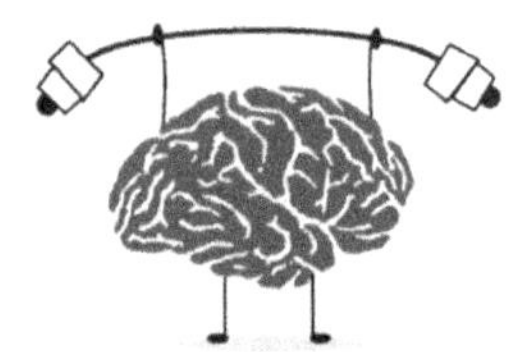

our **attention** muscle!

Do this with me **right now** –

(but only if it is ***safe*** for you to do so!)

- Sit comfortably.
- Set a timer for 1 minute. 
- Close your eyes or look down towards floor.
- As you breath **IN** – think… ***"My mind is calm"***
- As you breath **OUT** – think… ***"My body's relaxed"***

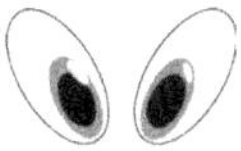

Use the video to help you practice…

Tinyurl.com/MindPushups

The Right Order

Now that you have some

of the **RIGHT TOOLS,**

It's time to understand

the **RIGHT ORDER.**

Let me ask you a  ...

How do you keep the tub

from overflowing?

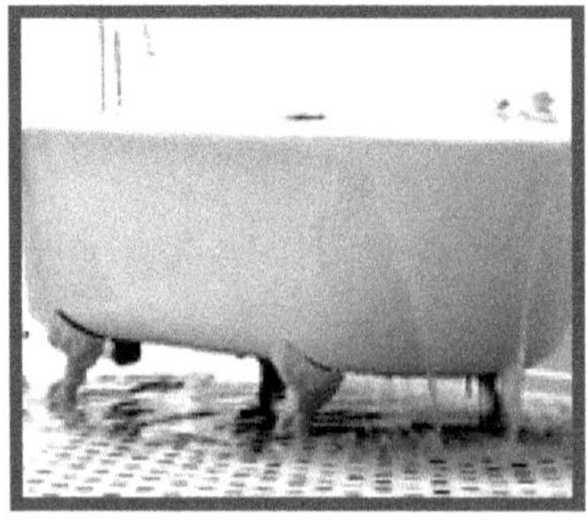

Most people I ask will say:

"Turn off the faucet."

But...

What happens if someone comes along

later and ***"turns it back on"?***

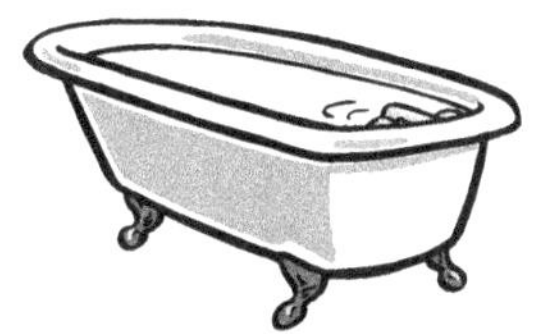

If it is close to the top –

It will **OVERFLOW!!!!**

So,

There are really **2** steps required

to keep the tub from overflowing:

1st - ***Turn Off*** the faucet.

2nd - ***Drain*** the tub!

Follow the Freedom Map™

By now you can 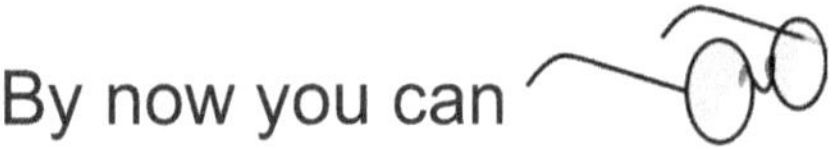

we can't just **Talk** or **Think**

our way out of stress!

We must **ACT**!

Introducing the **Freedom Map…**

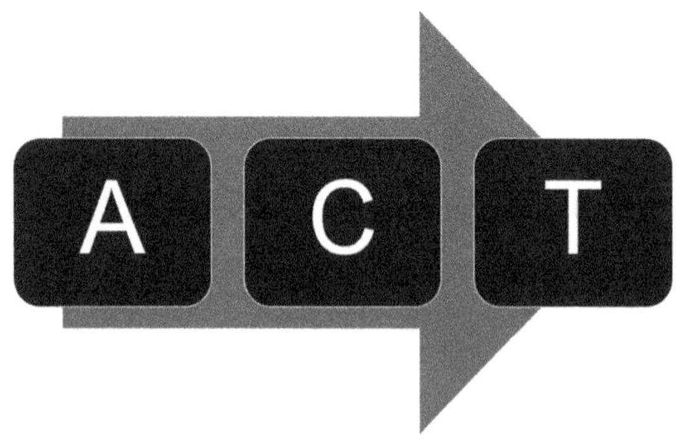

Following this map

will put you in *control!*

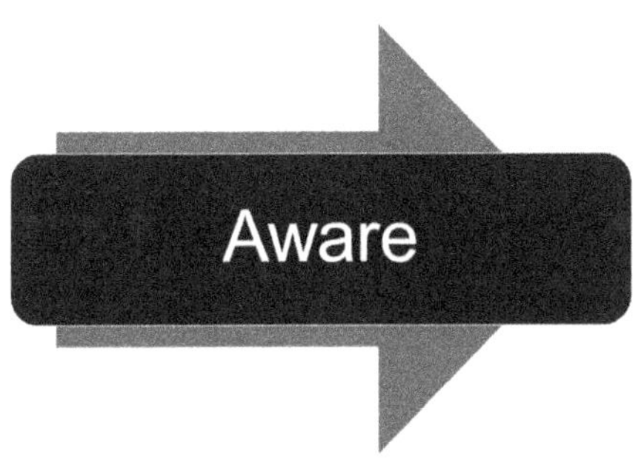

You MUST become aware of the

Changes or Situations

triggering your stress response.

We want to **avoid** them if we can…

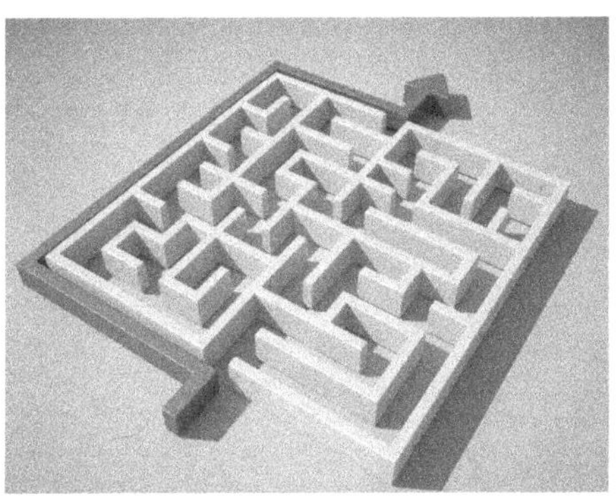

If we ***CAN'T***…. Keep following the map!

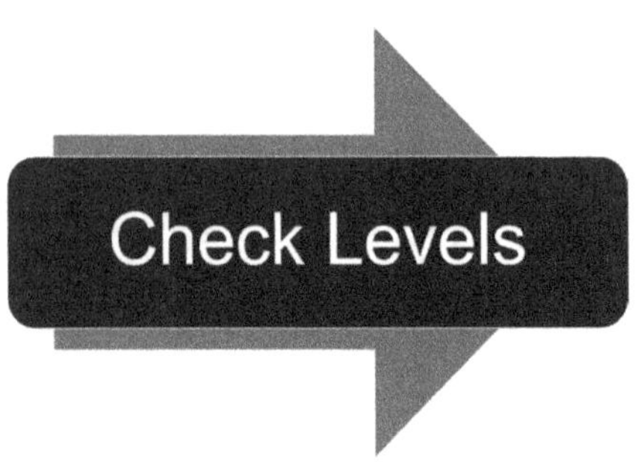

There are **2** ways you can do this:

1st Way:

Rate your stress level on a scale of

10 → 100

Low → High

2nd Way:

Pick which zone you're in:

green	yellow	red
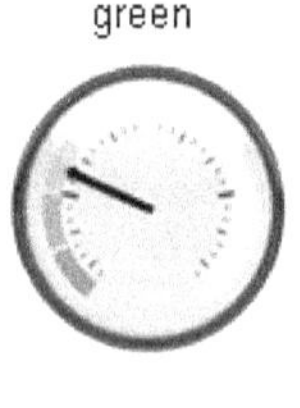	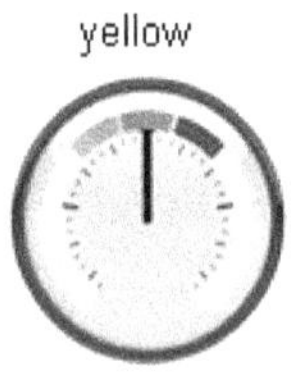	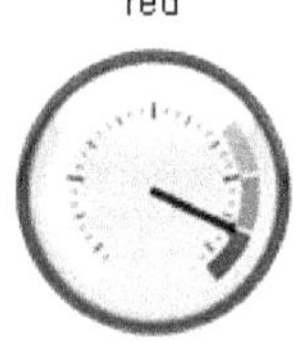
Safe	**Caution**	**Danger**

If you are a…

50 → 100

or in the

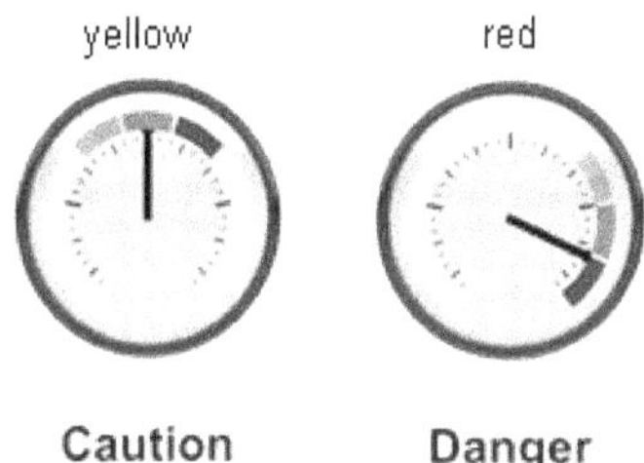

You **MUST** take immediate

action!

This is a sure sign the 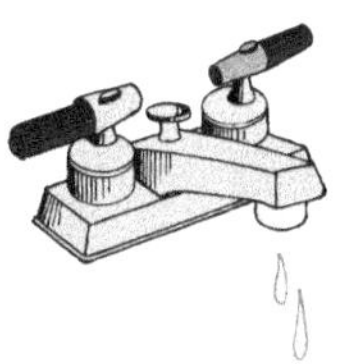 is on &

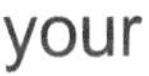

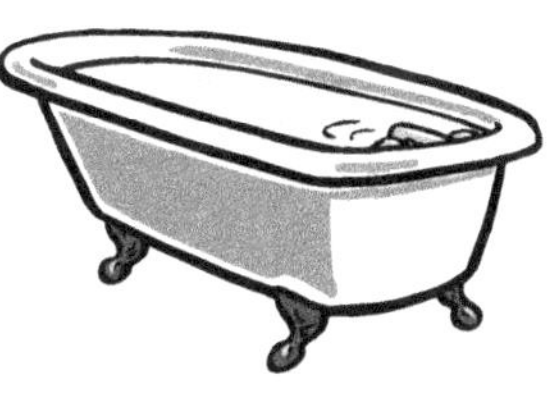

Is filling up fast!

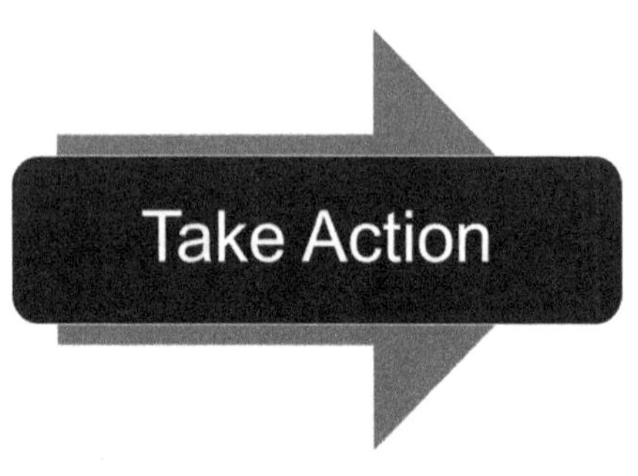

Now that you recognize your level

is ***BUILDING*** ***too high***

& we need to do something

BEFORE you:

Explode

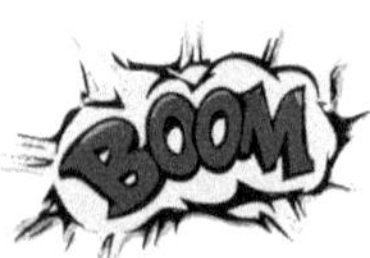

Implode

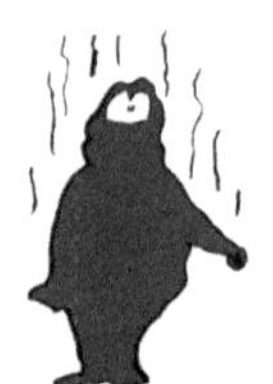

Combo

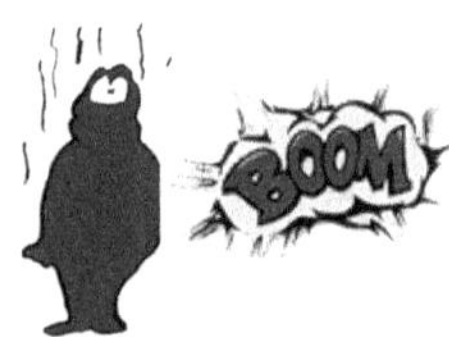

This brings us to the:

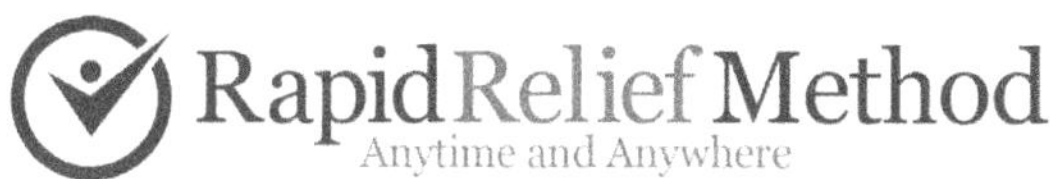

There are **2** simple steps to **SUCCESS:**

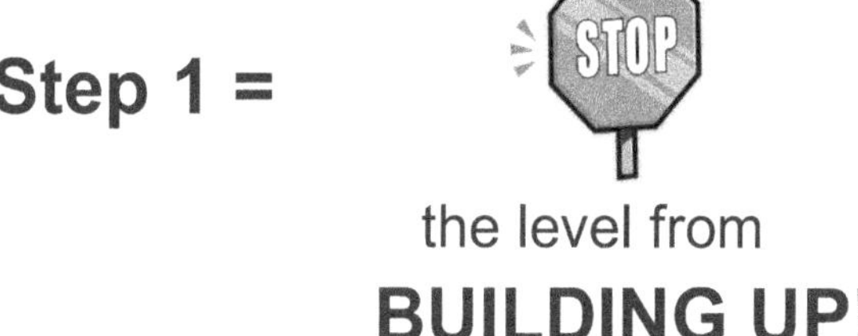

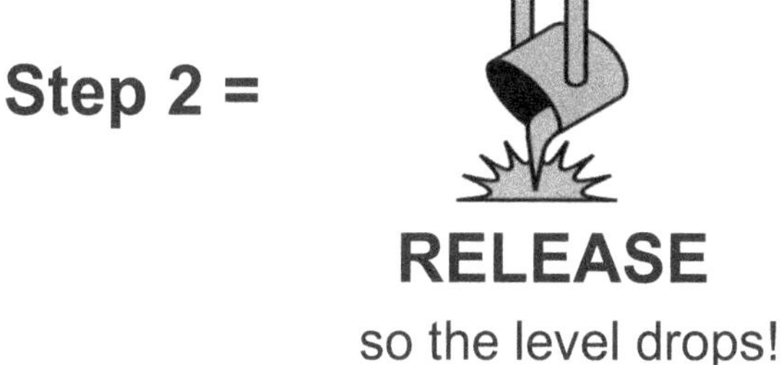

Each step must be done ***in order…***

Step 1 → Step 2

These tools below can used to STOP

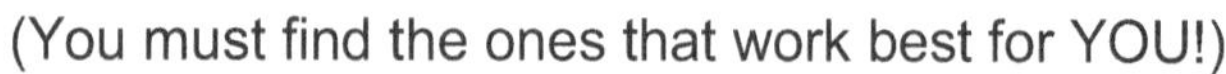

(You must find the ones that work best for YOU!)

Read

Count to 10

Step Away

Listen to Music

Breathing

Guided Imagery

Mind Pushups

Mantra / Quote

Prayer

Shower or bath

Aromatherapy

+ Self Talk

NOTICE:

STOP tools are passive, **no energy,**

and…

engage your brain!

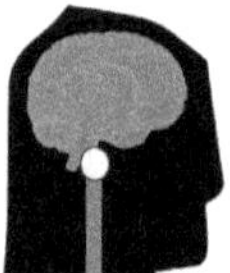

A Critical Point:

You MUST have tools that can be used…

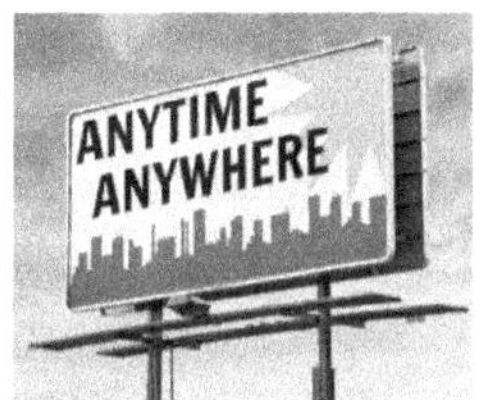

and no one knows!

There are **3** powerful 

tools we

ALWAYS have *with us…*

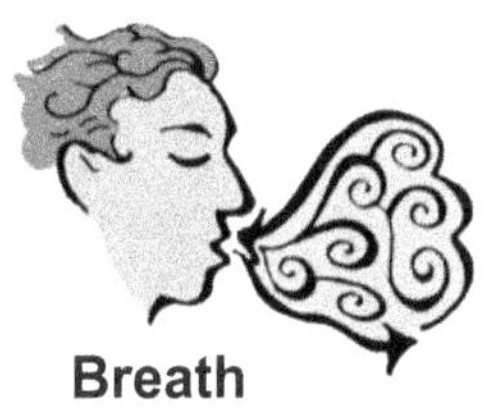

Breath

GOD GRANT ME THE SERENITY
TO ACCEPT THE THINGS
I CANNOT CHANGE,
COURAGE TO CHANGE
THE THINGS I CAN,
AND WISDOM
TO KNOW THE DIFFERENCE.

Mantra / Quote

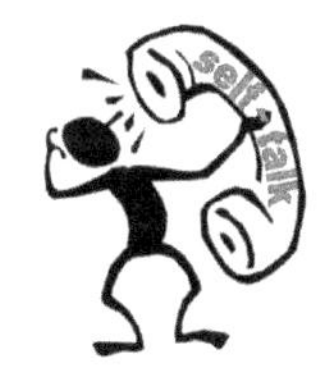

+ Self Talk

The tools below can be used to

(You must find the ones that work best for YOU!)

Talk	Coloring
Walk	Punching Bag
Write / Dump	Hobbies
Sing / Dance	Laughter
Clean	Gardening
Exercise	Ho, Ho, Ha, Ha

NOTICE:

RELEASE tools are active, **use energy,**

and…

engage your body!

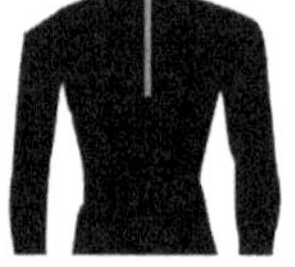

A Critical Point:

You MUST have tools that can be used…

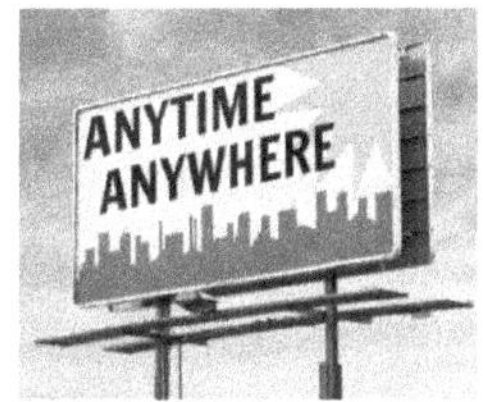

and no one knows!

Here are **3** powerful 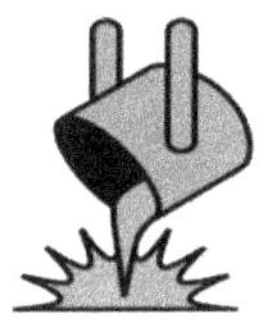 tools we

ALWAYS have *with us…*

Walk

Dump & Destroy

Talk

The method works because…

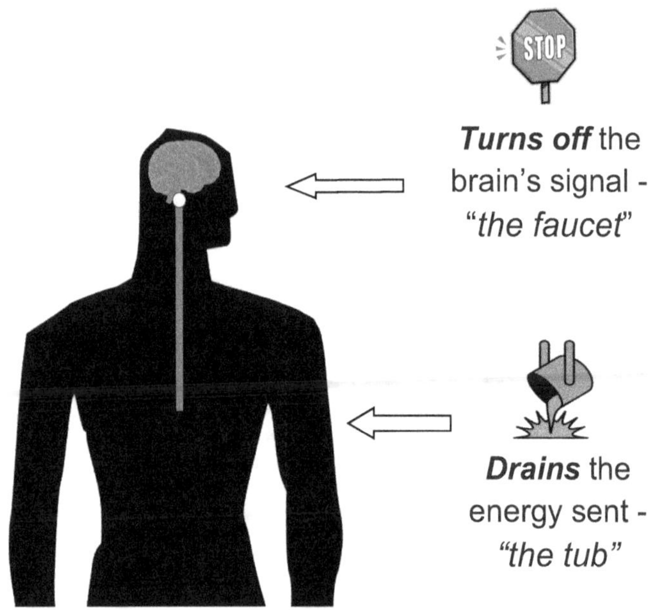

Although discovered 22 years ago…

it's only recent ***advances***

in neuroscience that help explain

why it works!

Stress Regulation

Because stress is inevitable….

just trying to "manage it" ***won't*** work!

Instead -

We need to *take action*

during the day to keep our stress at

the

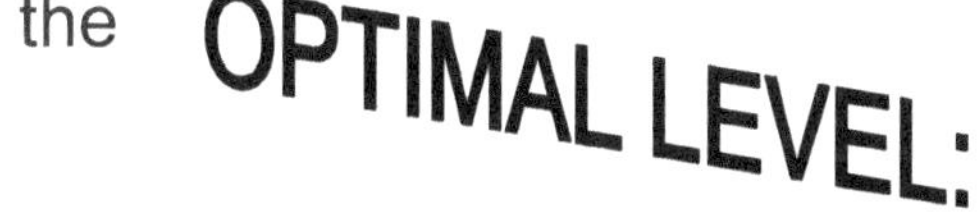

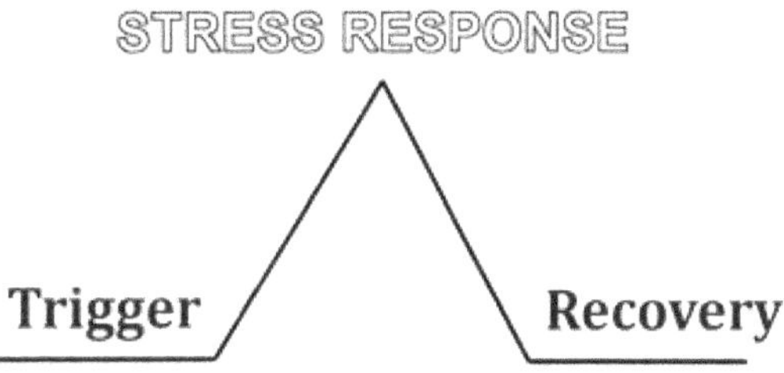

Stress happens…. **Stress Smarter!**

Proof It Works!

You *can* control **stress** & **anxiety**

if you will just **TAKE ACTION!**

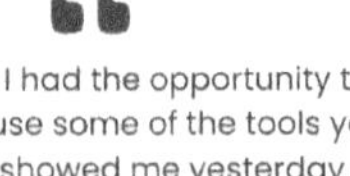

I had the opportunity to use some of the tools you showed me yesterday & it worked wonderfully. I'm so amazed!

"You held a captive audience with your energy & enthusiasm. You are great! I learned many tools I can learn to manage my stress."

Joanne Tavener-Smith
Wellness Coordinator
Office of Health & Wellness
New Jersey State Police

★★★★★

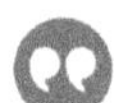

★★★★★

I appreciate the tools you provided! They will be valuable as I prepare for my upcoming procedure, and your support during my first therapy session has already made a positive impact. Thank you!

Best,
Helen

Wrap Up!

Could You

Be Living With

"Hidden Stress"?

Take the

"What's Your Hidden Stress Risk?" Quiz

Tinyurl.com/HiddenQuiz

What We Covered

Right at the start,

I introduced a **new way**

to 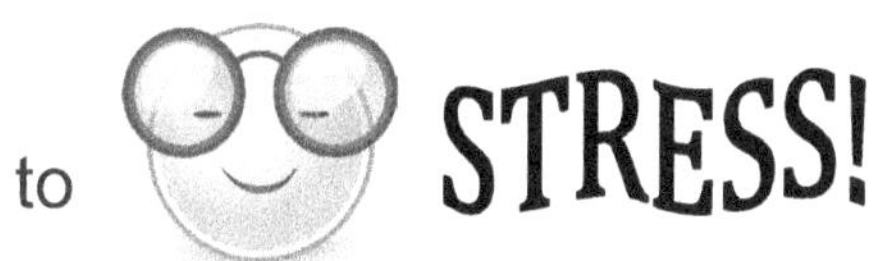

Life happens every day that

shakes us up!

Just like the pressure

BUILDS UP

in the bottle…

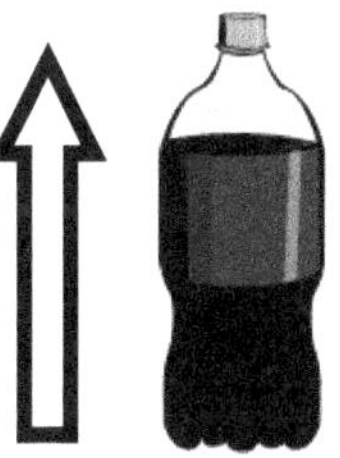

PRESSURE builds up *inside us!*

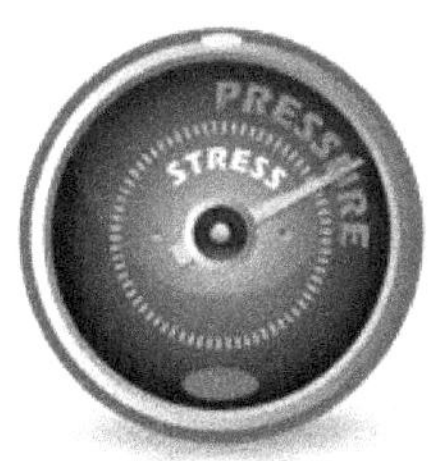

STRESS is…

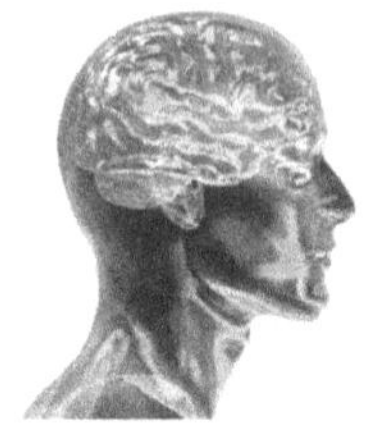

Our
Brain's
Survival
Mechanism

& YOU CAN'T STOP THE PROCESS!

It's ***"hardwired"*** to respond to

changes & situtations:

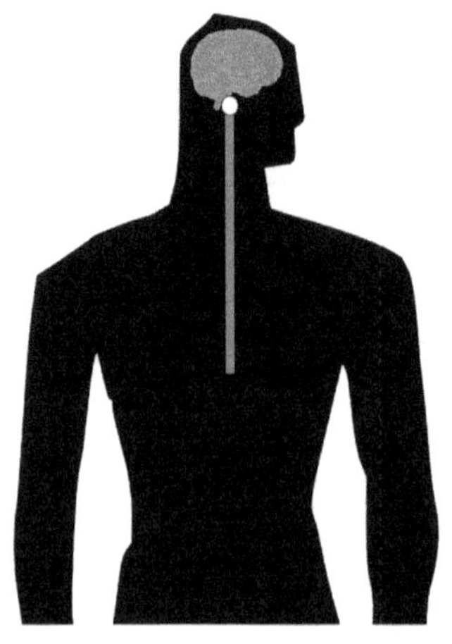

Defense Center
sends signals
& *energy to*

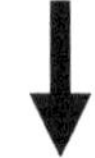

Our Body
We can't stop this –
Only MANAGE IT!

And…

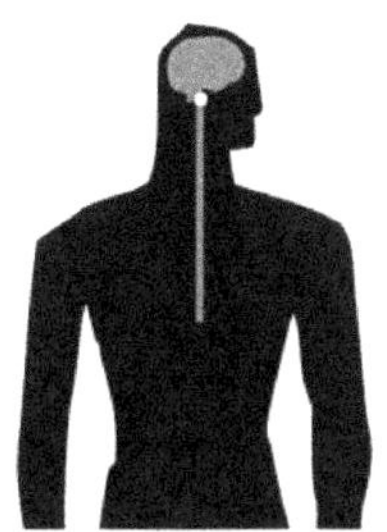

The Brain = Faucet

The Body = Tub

We can only hold so much before we…

Explode

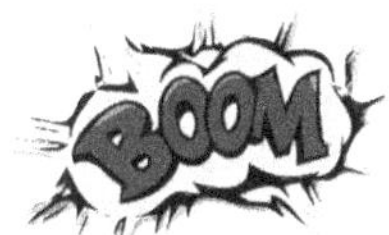

Implode

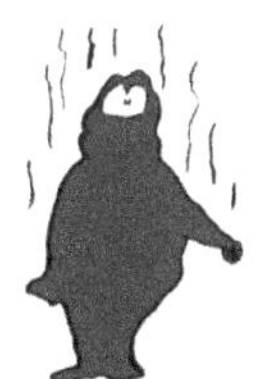

Combo

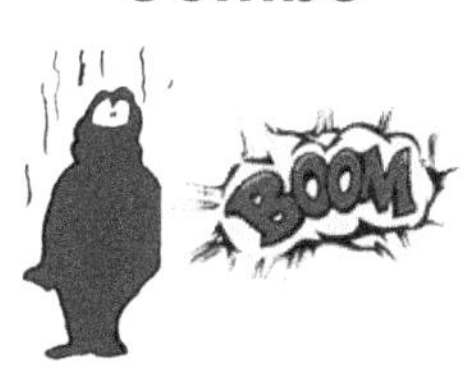

The good news is we can use the

RIGHT ***Tools*** in the **RIGHT** ***Order***

to take control!

The Right Tools:

- **Belly Breath**

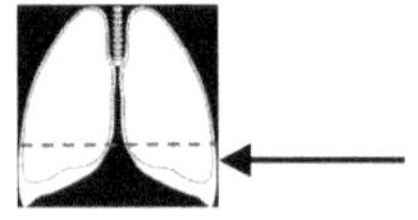

- **RESET Breath**

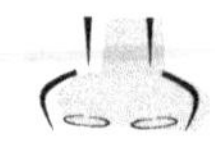

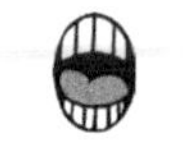

Slow 5 Slower 7

- **CALM Switch**

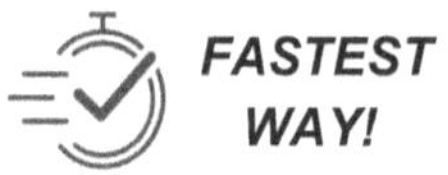

- **Dump n Destroy**

- **Mind Push-Up's**

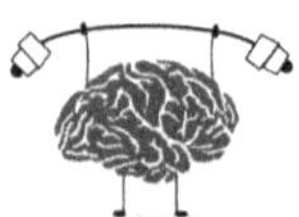

The Right Order:

Follow the Freedom Map!

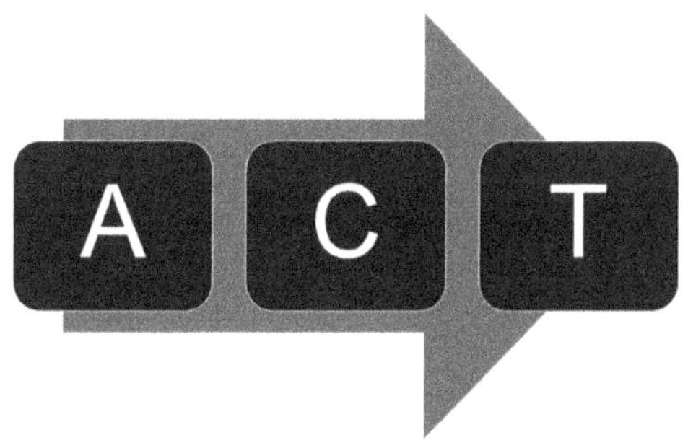

Aware (changes & situations)

Check (your stress level)

Take ***ACTION!*** (do 2 steps)

It's NOW up to **YOU** to…

use what you've learned!

Don't Miss This SPECIAL Offer!

Join Carol for the

Stress Smarter Masterclass

This 45-minute video training with Carol is a quick way to reinforce what you've learned!

ONLY $7

For A Limited Time...

SAVE $140

Tinyurl.com/bycarol

Need More Tools?!

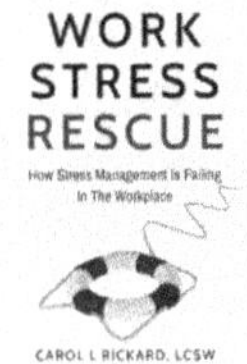

Work can be a challenging place! This gives you so many more tools to ensure your success in the workplace.

And Carol has written more "tool" books!

If you need help:

- ✓ Losing weight
- ✓ Dealing with anger
- ✓ Managing health issues
- ✓ Beginning meditation
- ✓ Practicing self-care

Take a look at the next few pages...

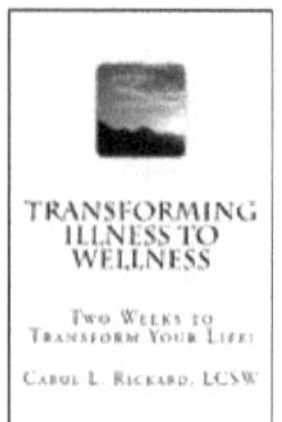

Chronic illness doesn't exclude you from having wellness. Get a blueprint to follow for taking back control of your health!

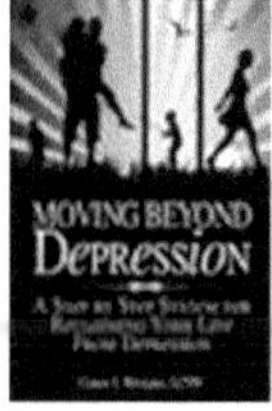

Are you sick & tired of feeling sick & tired? This is a step by step system for reclaiming your life from depression.

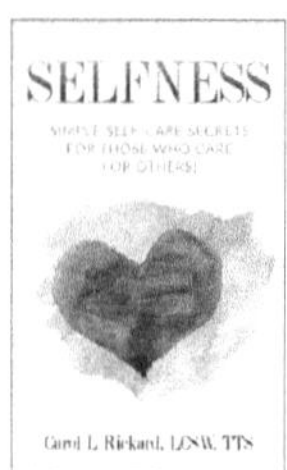

Self-care is often forgotten in this busy world. Carol offers simple and practical strategies to fit in to your busy life!

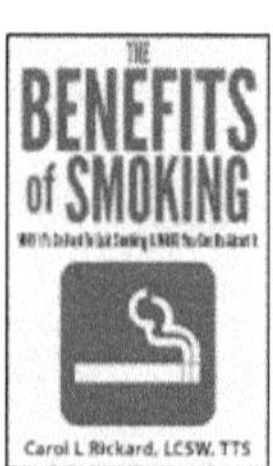

No – this is not promoting smoking! Instead, it provides the knowledge & the 'tools' to finally "Kick Cigarettes Butts"!

Available: amazon.com/author/carolrickard

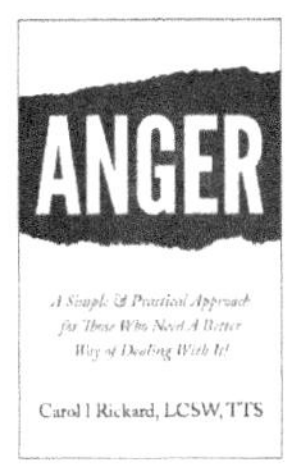

ANGER - one of the most powerful emotions there is. Learn how to manage it instead of it managing you!

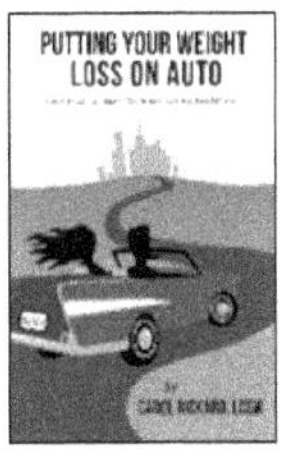

Losing weight doesn't have to be complicated! Learn the *7 Laws of Lasting Weight Loss* a car can teach us.
Guaranteed to work!

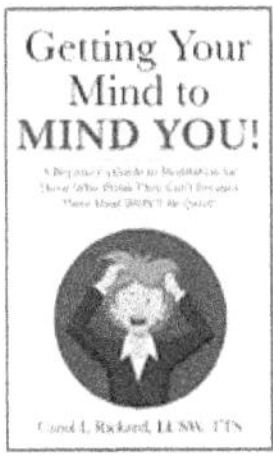

Your mind *is not* supposed to be quiet! Learn how mediation really works & change your life forever!

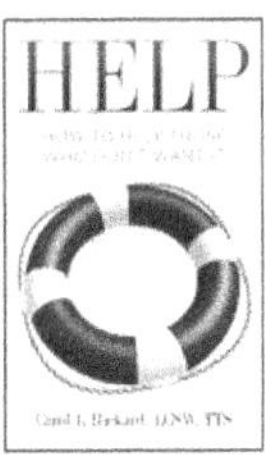

Do you find yourself struggling with what to say or how to help someone you care about? Learn how to say it & what to

Available: amazon.com/author/carolrickard

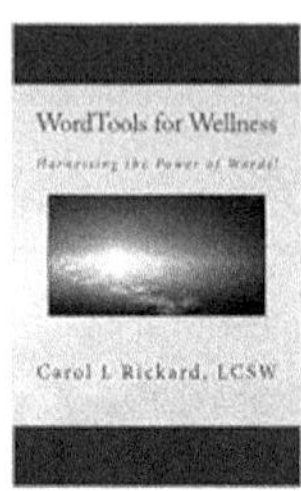

WordTools

What are words tools?
They are acronyms with purpose & meaning!

They are officially called *Artinyms*™, which is Sanskrit for "describe".

On the back of each wordtool is a question for you to answer should you choose to!

We have **4 different versions:**

Wellness Vol. 1 & 2, ***Self-Esteem*** Vol. 1 & 2
Business Vol. 1 & 2, ***Athletes*** Vol. 1

Examples:

The
Only
Day
Afforded
You!

A
Deliberate
Adjustment
Providing
Transformation

Daringly
Recognize
Experiences
As
Mine

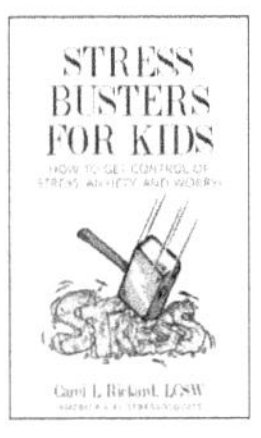

NEW RELEASE!!!!
Kid these days have to deal with so much stress. This makes sure they have the tools to succeed!!

We have three different versions of adult stress books because life circumstances can be different for each.

Choose the one that ***best fits*** your situation!

Caregiver

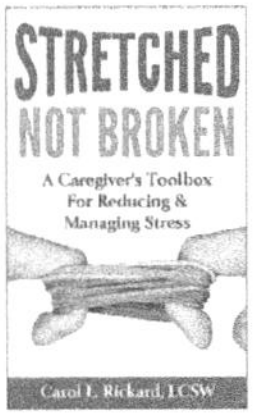

Research has shown caregivers are the MOST vulnerable. Learn quick, simple, practical tools for reducing and managing it.

Stress Eater

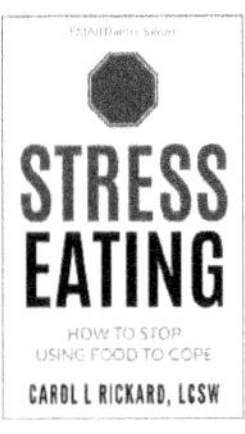

Do you find yourself eating when under stress? Get the tools & knowledge needed to break away from any old habits.

General

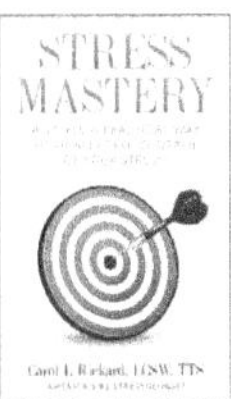

STRESS… It's all around us and NOT getting any less! Get the system Carol has taught to 1,000's & finally take control!

This series of books introduces Carol's proprietary method™ that you learned about in this book! Each version has added chapters geared towards that **specific audience.**

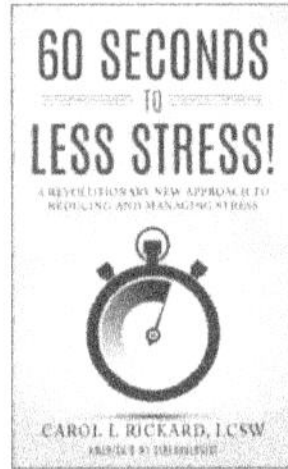

General Audience - This is the book that started the series! You'll learn the system that lets you finally take control of stress!

Brides

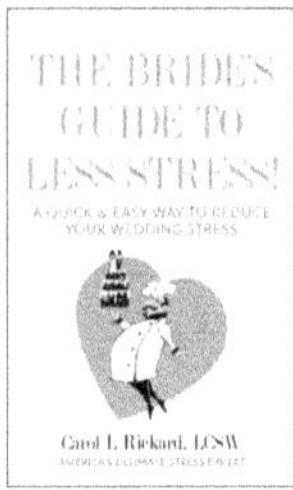

Nurses

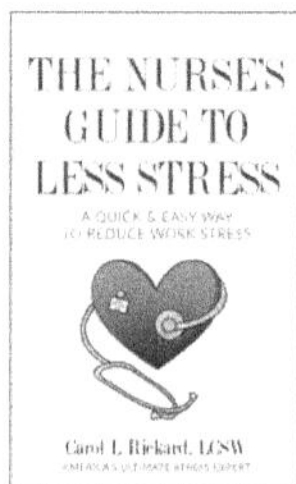

Caregivers

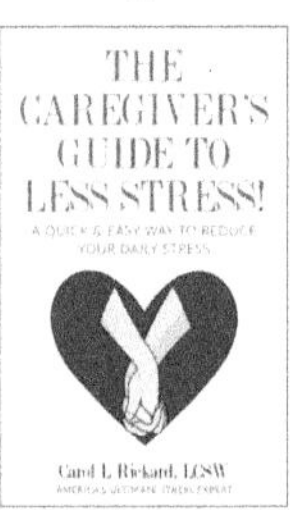

Teachers

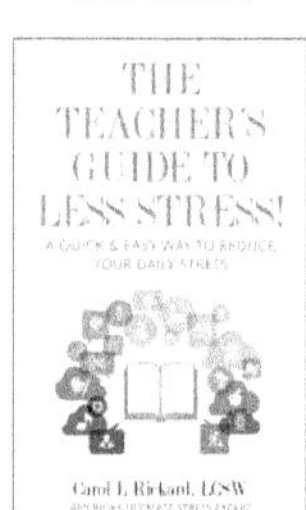

Available: amazon.com/author/carolrickard

Don't Miss This SPECIAL Offer!

Join Carol for the

Stress Smarter Masterclass

This 45-minute video training with Carol is a quick way to reinforce what you've learned!

ONLY $7

For A Limited Time…

SAVE $140

Tinyurl.com/bycarol

About The Author

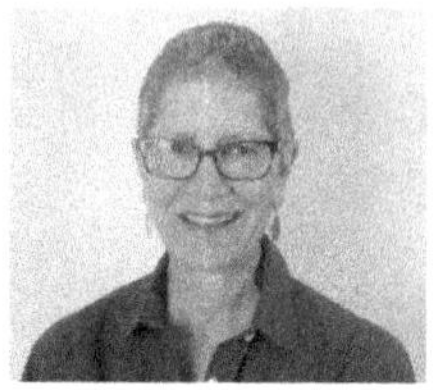

Carol Rickard, LCSW is a distinguished health and wellness expert dedicated to equipping individuals with the tools necessary to recognize and effectively manage stress. With over 30 years of clinical practice, Carol has developed a groundbreaking method that enables people to alleviate stress and anxiety in just seconds.

Her innovative approach extends to her recently developed quiz, designed to help individuals uncover "Hidden Stress" that may be impacting their mental health. This free 30-second quiz, titled "What's Your Hidden Stress Risk?" offers a quick and insightful assessment, guiding users to better understand their unique stress profiles.

As a stage III cancer survivor, Carol intimately understands the urgency of having effective coping mechanisms when life takes unexpected turns. She has authored over 25 books on stress management, sharing her expert knowledge and practical strategies to help thousands lead healthier, more resilient lives.

Her award-winning books, coupled with a nationally syndicated television show, have transformed the lives of many by providing real-world solutions to everyday challenges.

Speaking:

Carol is available to do both live and virtual speaking events. Contact her to get more details.

To Contact Carol:

Please feel free to reach out if you have questions or comments. She'd love to hear how this book has helped you!

Email:

Carol@CarolRickard.com

Connect with Carol on:

Linkedin.com/in/CarolLRickard

Facebook.com/CarolLRickard

Youtube.com/@CarolLRickard

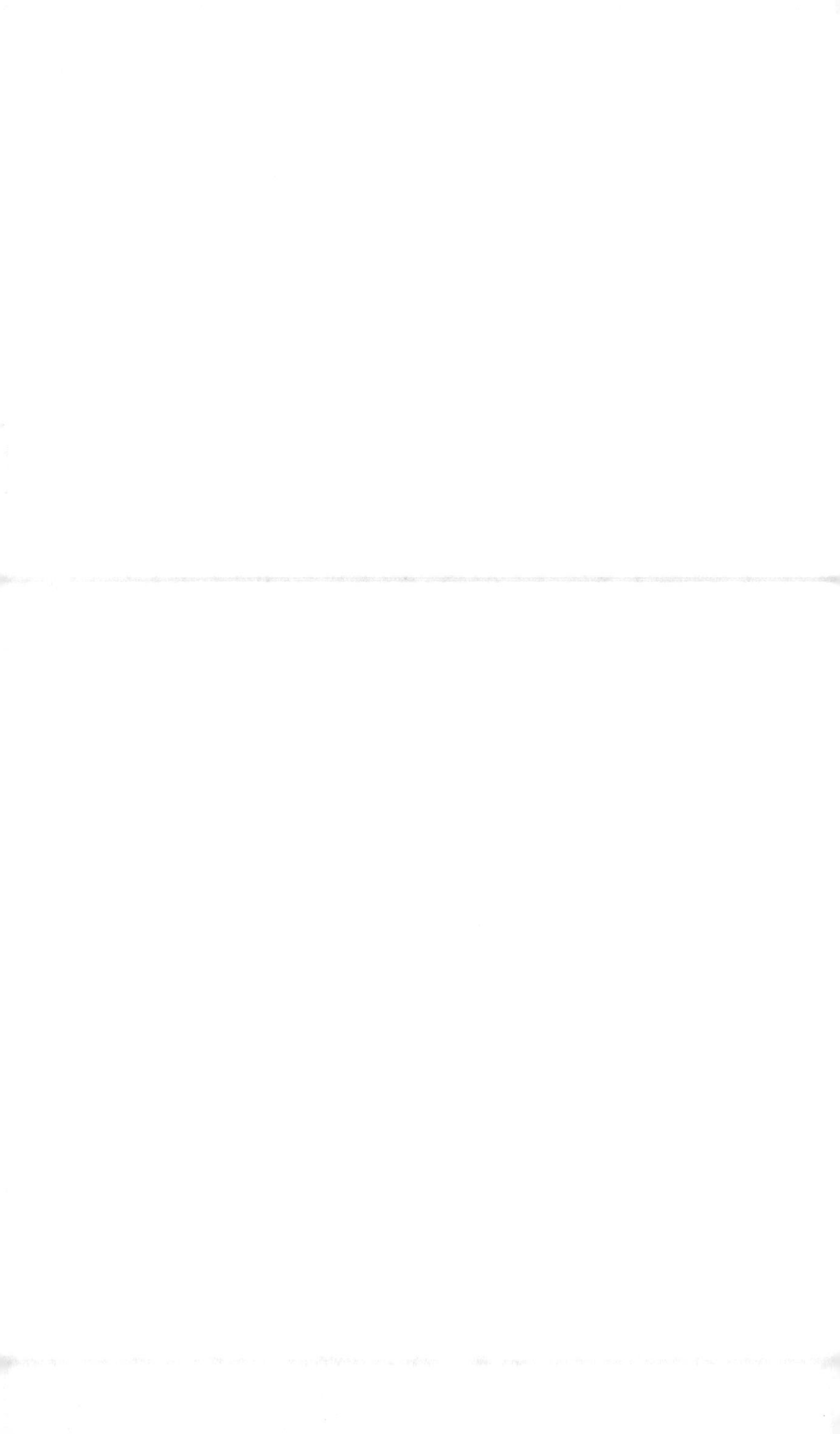